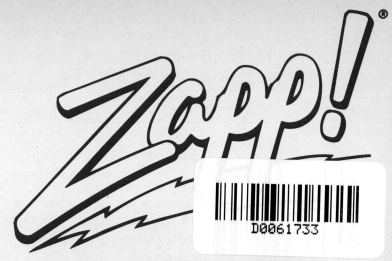

EMPOWERMENT IN HEALTH CARE

HOW TO IMPROVE PATIENT CARE, INCREASE EMPLOYEE JOB SATISFACTION, AND LOWER HEALTH CARE COSTS

WILLIAM C. BYHAM, PH.D.,

WITH JEFF COX, KATHY HARPER SHOMO, AND SHARYN MATERNA

FAWCETT COLUMBINE • NEW YORK

To my wife, Carolyn,
who has kept the Zapp! in my life
for more than 25 years.

© Copyright 1993 by Development Dimensions International, Inc.

All rights reserved under International and Pan-American Copyright Conventions. No part of this book may be reproduced or utilized in any form or by any means, electronic or mechanical, including photocopying, recording, or by any information storage and retrieval system, without permission in writing from Development Dimensions International. Published in the United States by Ballantine Books, a division of Random House, Inc., New York, and simultaneously in Canada by Random House of Canada Limited, Toronto.

Library of Congress Catalog Card Number: 93-90240

ISBN: 0-449-90885-2

Text design by Holly Johnson

Manufactured in the United States of America

First Edition: June 1993

10 9 8 7 6 5 4 3 2 1

More praise for

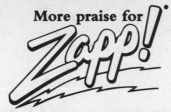

EMPOWERMENT IN HEALTH CARE

"The advice is practical, and the book is easy to read and very enjoyable. All the key steps for quality implementation and self-analysis of management style are presented in an entertaining manner. I highly recommend the book for all health care managers and clinicians. The lessons presented are critical for those seeking improvement of the health care system."

> —Ellen Gaucher
> Senior Associate Director
> University of Michigan Hospitals

"Bill Byham has woven some of the key values, principles, tools, and techniques of Total Quality Management into a hospital tale that is entertaining, believable, and learnable."

> —Frank V. Murphy
> President and C.E.O.
> Morton Plant Hospital

"*Zapp! Empowerment in Health Care* presents the essence of quality health services management in a delightfully entertaining and informative manner. All of my students will read this book . . . and you should, too."

> —Joseph F. Constable, Ph.D.
> Program Director
> Health Services Management
> Robert Morris College

CONTENTS

OTHER BOOKS ON EMPOWERMENT
BY WILLIAM C. BYHAM

Empowered Teams: Creating Self-Directed Work Groups That Improve Quality, Productivity, and Participation with Richard S. Wellins and Jeanne M. Wilson.

Shogun Management: How North Americans Can Thrive in Japanese Companies with George Dixon.

Zapp! in Education with Jeff Cox and Kathy Harper Shomo.

Zapp! The Lightning of Empowerment with Jeff Cox.

For information on any of these books, write or call us at Development Dimensions International, World Headquarters—Pittsburgh, 1225 Washington Pike, Bridgeville, PA 15017-2838, (412) 257-2277, between 8:00 A.M. and 5:00 P.M. EST.

PREFACE

Why Should You Read This Book?

That is a fair question. Why should a serious, rational adult take time to read a fable about problems and achievements of health care providers, hospital administrators, and patients in a make-believe hospital?

One reason to read this book is the need to improve the quality of patient care in American hospitals. Unfortunately, while medical costs have continued to rise, patients report that they receive less individual attention than ever before. Many treatments that formerly involved overnight stays now are handled on an outpatient basis, resulting in significantly less follow-up care. And even those patients who remain in hospitals for extended periods of time often complain that their doctors and nurses are too busy tending to the technical aspects of their care—or simply too busy period—to provide much-needed attention to their personal needs.

A second reason to read this book is that many health care providers feel frustrated and disillusioned in jobs that they expected to find fulfilling. They feel that they do not have enough time to do a quality job of caring for their patients. They cut corners, see waste, and think they can't do anything to change the situation. They feel they are unappreciated and their skills underused. These feelings lead to low morale, staff turnover, and disenchantment with job opportunities in health care.

The third reason is the spiraling cost of health care. Currently, 14 percent of the United States GNP is spent on health care; this figure is expected to reach 18 percent by the year 2000. People at every level agree that something has to be done—and quickly. America's disproportionately high health care costs are hurting our domestic economy because products are priced higher, which is a great disadvantage when U.S. organizations compete with companies in other countries. As government organizations and private companies pressure hospitals, physicians, other providers, and third-party payers to cut costs and improve efficiency, many are finding it difficult to meet these goals.

The thesis of this book is that greater empowerment (job identification and ownership) of health care employees can lead to better patient care, greater job satisfaction, and lower health care costs. This is because empowerment energizes the people who are closest to the patients and the technology to continuously look for ways to provide high-quality patient care and improve processes. The accumulation of ideas—both large and small—from many people will result in better patient care and operational efficiencies.

Empowered people see themselves as meaningful, respected, and appreciated individuals who are recognized for their ideas and contributions. They see their jobs as interesting, challenging, and rewarding. They realize that empowerment enables them to "make a difference" by meeting patients' personal and practical needs as well as organizational needs. Empowered people are involved and committed to their work, and they gain satisfaction from their successes. For empowered individuals, caring for others and making the organization work better are two sides of the same coin. One cannot be achieved without the other.

This book was written for the health care leader who wants to provide an environment conducive to empowerment and for everyone else in the organization who must seize the opportunities afforded by empowerment. It is designed to help health care professionals understand, at a fundamental level, what empowerment is, why it is important, and how its principles can be used in health care organizations everywhere.

Zapp! Empowerment in Health Care is an adaptation of *Zapp! The Lightning of Empowerment*, which focuses on life in a corporate setting. Because of the original book's tremendous success—and the great interest shown by health care professionals—we have developed a variation of this story to show how the same concepts can be used in health care organizations. Based on Development Dimensions International's (DDI's) experience with more than 500 hospital clients in the United States, Canada, and the United Kingdom, we expanded the contents to cover issues, such as process improvement and organizational structure, that are particularly pertinent to today's health care organizations. We sincerely hope you will find *Zapp! Empowerment in Health Care* as helpful to you as the first *Zapp!* book has been for business professionals.

Why did we write the book in the style of a fable? Because even the best ideas are of small value unless communicated well. *Zapp! Empowerment in Health Care* is written the way it is so that an abstract concept can be visualized in action—in lively but meaningful terms. We wanted the book to be easy to understand, yet challenging to the imagination. Fable or not, this is a realistic, practical book. After you have read it, you will know what to do to be empowered and to empower others, and you will have a sound basis for beginning formal training in empowerment skills.

So enjoy *Zapp! Empowerment in Health Care*. And, most important, learn about a concept that is vital to personal and professional success—a concept that might, in fact, hold the key to our national health care challenge.

Pittsburgh, Pennsylvania

PART I

Situation Normal

I

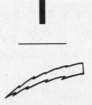

Once upon a time, in a magic land called America, there lived a normal nurse named Florence Knight. Her friends called her Flo.

Flo worked as a registered nurse at Normal Medical Center, a 350-bed community hospital located in Normalburg, U.S.A. For years, Normal Medical Center had operated as a good hospital and had gained the respect of the community it served. Many of the town's leading citizens had been treated there—some had even been born there—and the townspeople had high regard for the hospital and its staff.

As you might expect, just about everything was normal at Normal, including the understanding of who was normally supposed to do what:

The Board of Directors did the thinking.
Hospital administrators did the talking.
Physicians made all decisions about patient care.
Support services did all the supporting—and
    anything else they were asked to do.

Nurses told patients what to do.

And the patients did what they were told—well, most of the time.

That was the way it had always been—ever since the town's foreparents had built the hospital—and so everybody just assumed that was the way it should always be.

Flo was your normal type of nurse. She was well educated. She enjoyed caring for her patients. She handled the reports her nursing supervisor asked her to complete. And at the end of the day, she dragged herself home, tired and frustrated that she couldn't have done more for her patients.

When friends or family asked how she liked nursing, Flo would say, "Oh, it's all right, I guess. Not very exciting, but I guess that's normal. Anyway, it's a job and the pay is OK."

In truth, being a nurse at Normal Medical Center was not very satisfying for Flo, although she was not sure why. Her schedule wasn't bad. The benefits were fine. The other nurses were well educated and dedicated. They were all considered to be good nurses, although no one really knew what that meant. The patients were as pleasant as could be expected under the circumstances. Yet, something seemed to be missing.

But Flo figured there wasn't much she could do to change things at the hospital. After all, she reasoned, who would even bother to listen? So she kept her thoughts to herself, and just did what she was told.

Flo worked on the Medical-Surgical unit of Normal Medical Center. One day, on her way back to the Med-Surg unit from lunch, Flo happened to be thinking about one of her patients and . . . well, she was simply *Zapped* by an idea so original and so full of promise that her head nearly exploded with excitement.

"Yes! That's it!" exclaimed Flo, to the shock of all the Normal nurses around her.

In her excitement, Flo totally forgot that probably nobody would listen, and she ran down the hall to explain her idea to the Med-Surg nursing supervisor, JoAnn Mode.

Flo found JoAnn busy, doing what she normally did. She was telling everybody what to do as she worried about four patient problems she had to deal with, lab results that were several hours late, and the monthly meeting of all the unit supervisors being held that afternoon. As JoAnn was scribbling a memo to her staff, she received an urgent call from the director of nursing.

JoAnn's boss, Mary Ellen Krabofski, was quite upset. That morning she had had to deal with several problems in other units. In Obstetrics, there had been three emergency deliveries, just as one shift was ending and another was beginning. One of the mothers was very upset because her regular doctor was out of town, which meant that Baby Andrew had to be delivered by "a total stranger." To make matters worse, the new father had fainted just as the baby's head popped out, causing more than one physician to think back to the good old days when there was only the mother to worry about in the delivery room—not the father, too.

And now the new father was upset because he had missed the big event—and embarrassed himself big time. The attending physician refused to deal with the situation, so it had become Mary Ellen's problem. This had put her in a bad mood for the entire day.

Later in the morning, Mary Ellen had received another upsetting call. This time, the complaint was from the nursing supervisor in Pediatrics, who was having difficulty with one of the unit nurses. Sandy had excellent clinical skills but often was rude to patients, their families, and other staff members. This morning, during a rush period, Sandy had been extremely abrupt with the mother of a young patient. As a result of her temper and some inconsiderate remarks, the parents had decided to ask their pediatrician about the possibility of moving their daughter from Normal Medical Center to another hospital.

And just now, a woman had called to complain about how long it was taking JoAnn's nurses to answer her husband's call bell. That's when Mary Ellen decided to call JoAnn.

"JoAnn, I want you to start cracking the whip over there," Mary Ellen told her. "Employee apathy is evident in your unit. And our patients aren't exactly thrilled with Med-Surg. Just this week, I've received two letters from unhappy patients and their families. And now this phone call."

"But I do crack the whip," JoAnn responded. "Every chance I get."

"Well," said Mary Ellen, "whatever you're doing, it isn't good enough. The C.E.O. wants all of us to do better. He says the federal and state regulations are strict and they're getting stricter. Funding is short and it's getting shorter. Admissions are low and they're getting lower. Doctor and patient complaints are numerous and they're getting more numerous. So you'd better do something fast—or else!"

"But what can I do?" JoAnn asked in desperation.

"Make doctors happy, JoAnn! Make patients happy! Improve employee morale! Find ways to save money! And, above all, do a good job!"

"Right. Got it," said JoAnn.

"Then get to it!"

They both hung up. That was when JoAnn saw Flo standing off to the side, eagerly waiting to talk about her idea.

"So talk," JoAnn sighed.

As Flo explained her idea, which was so original and full of promise, JoAnn continued what she was already doing.

"How are you coming with the patient reports you're supposed to have finished by the end of the shift?" asked JoAnn, ignoring Flo's idea and enthusiasm.

"I'll finish the reports. But what about my idea?" asked Flo, still excited.

"It doesn't sound to me like the normal way to do things," said JoAnn. "And besides, don't you think that if the idea was *really* good, one of the vendors that supplies us with all our high-tech equipment would have thought of it?"

At that moment, Flo was tempted to tell JoAnn that specialists outside the hospital didn't know everything, and that furthermore . . .

But, being normal, Flo didn't tell JoAnn anything. She just nodded and went back to work. And JoAnn went back to telling everybody what to do and worrying about the work that had to be finished that afternoon.

By the end of the shift, Flo's reports were not completed. She left them on the desk and headed for the parking lot with the other nurses. And JoAnn, feeling a sense of defeat, sat down at her desk and worried about Mary Ellen Krabofski.

2

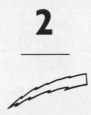

One thing to JoAnn Mode's credit, she was organized. Over the years, she had developed the habit of writing things down, and all this jotting and scribbling had evolved into a notebook she kept at her desk. JoAnn got out her notebook and wrote down the problem as she saw it.

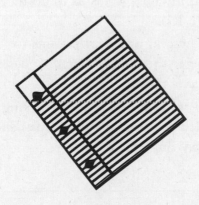

JoAnn Mode's Notebook

The problem as I see it:

- Government regulators and health care consumers want more for less.
- The Board of Directors wants more for less.
- The Chief Executive Officer and Chief Operating Officer want more for less.
- And my boss wants us to do more with less.
- Because in order for patients to receive the quality care they deserve, it takes more.
- But we don't seem to be making much progress in cutting costs and improving efficiency.

Then she made a list of all the things she thought might be wrong.

JoAnn Mode's Notebook

What is wrong:

- Hardly anybody gets excited about their jobs anymore.
- The things they do get excited about are outside of work.
- My nurses and aides care about their patients, but they spend half their time doing paperwork.
- My staff wants to provide the best quality of patient care possible, but they don't have the time or energy to do more than the bare minimum.
- I talk about being more efficient and what happens? Lots of blank looks.
- It seems that when anybody shows exceptional competence, the only reward is more work. Most of the credit, recognition, and pride go to the doctors.

Notebook ▤ (cont'd)

- Nobody takes any more responsibility for problems than they have to. If the patients and their families aren't happy, it's *my* problem.

- All day it's as if everyone is operating in overdrive, but only the bare minimum gets done.

- We all do our jobs according to the rules so we won't get yelled at or disciplined—even when the rules don't fit a particular situation.

- The general attitude is: Don't try to change anything. It's a waste of time.

- Whenever I try to motivate my nurses or aides, the results (if any) are short lived.

- Everyone cares about improving, but they're all afraid of change. (Me, too, if I'm honest about it.)

Of course, not all these things were true all the time. JoAnn Mode knew there were individual differences among people. But overall, that was how it seemed to her.

Then she started a new page, the page where she would come up with a brilliant solution that would solve the entire problem quickly and easily.

She sat there.

And sat there.

And sat there some more.

But no brilliant solution was forthcoming. Finally, she wrote . . .

JoAnn Mode's Notebook

The solution:

How should I know? I'm just a nursing supervisor.

What am I going to do now?

- Wait for more regulations from the government and other agencies.
- Wait for senior management to come up with a brilliant solution.
- Think about a career change.

Why?

Because at the rate things are going, Normal Medical Center is in for trouble—and all the health care providers in our community won't be far behind!

Then she closed her notebook, locked it away in her desk, and headed home. It had not been a good day.

3

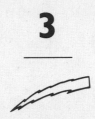

Of course, JoAnn Mode soon forgot about Flo's idea. But Flo did not. And, because of that, something very *ab*normal began to take place.

It so happened that an old research lab was located at the far end of the Medical–Surgical wing, a place where JoAnn normally did not venture because it was not officially a part of the unit.

This allowed Flo a place to work on her new invention. Soon after coming up with her idea, Flo found herself going into work early or staying late in order to work on it. Instead of chatting with the other nurses on her lunch hour, she thought about her idea and started making sketches. Then she talked with a friend of hers who was a biomedical engineer at Normal Medical Center. Together they worked on Flo's creation, using discarded equipment from the hospital lab and an old computer Flo brought in from home.

Weeks passed. And, little by little, Flo perfected the

invention—a new piece of hospital equipment that she called:

Flo-Vision

The other nurses noticed a change in Flo. The doctors noticed, too. She seemed to have more energy. She seemed more productive than ever. Patients commented on how pleasant she was to them. Flo seemed *happy*.

Of course, Flo encountered many setbacks and made a multitude of mistakes. But she stuck with it. She was determined to create something that would help health care organizations and patients everywhere. Finally, one morning after Flo had worked the night shift, she went to the old research lab and soldered the last wires into the control panel. The Flo-Vision was finished. Flo was pleased and proud.

Naturally, she just had to try it out. So she connected the wire leads to an old chair she had found, sat down, flipped a few switches, and typed in a command.

A high-pitched whine began to emanate from the innards of the strange machine. The work area began to pulsate with an unearthly light. Flo gripped the arms of her chair, grinned with anticipation—and vanished in a powerful flash.

Several hours later, JoAnn needed to know something about a report Flo had submitted. When her assistant nursing supervisor, Phyllis, explained that Flo hadn't gone home yet, JoAnn set out to look for her.

On her way down the hall, JoAnn heard some loud noises coming from one of the patient rooms. She decided to find out what was going on.

Inside Room 311, the lab technician was arguing with Mr. Bentley, a big, surly man who was recovering from recent gallbladder surgery.

"Just stick out your arm!" bellowed Louise, the lab technician.

"No! You aren't getting any more blood from me. And that's that!" yelled Mr. Bentley.

"You're on my list. That means I take blood," said Louise, matter-of-factly preparing her needle and tubes, her back to the patient.

"I said 'no!' and I mean 'no!' " repeated Mr. Bentley, who now was sitting with his arms crossed, staring at the lab technician in obvious defiance.

JoAnn decided that if she didn't intervene, things could only get worse. So she stepped into the room, forcing a smile as she spoke: "What's the problem, Mr. Bentley?"

"Attila the Nurse here thinks she's going to stick me with more needles—and she isn't! My doctor discharged me this morning, and he didn't say anything about anybody taking more blood from me. As soon as my wife gets here, I'm going home. And the sooner, the better."

JoAnn turned to Louise and asked to see her list of patients. Sure enough, Mr. Bentley's name was there.

"Well, Mr. Bentley, you are on the lab technician's list. And you weren't on my list of patients to be discharged today. Let me go to the nurses' station and call your doctor. I'm sure we can straighten this out very quickly."

Then, to Louise, JoAnn added, "Why don't you see to the other patients on this floor while I check with Dr. Lee. After you've finished with the other patients, stop by my office to see what I've found out about Mr. Bentley."

"Fine," muttered Louise, who noisily collected all her equipment and left the room in a huff.

"Mr. Bentley, just sit tight. I'll be right back," promised JoAnn.

Back at the nurses' station, a quick check with Dr. Lee confirmed JoAnn's guess: Mr. Bentley was doing well enough to be discharged two days earlier than scheduled. But because the new discharge date hadn't been communicated to the hematology lab, Louise still had Mr. Bentley on her list for drawing blood today.

JoAnn thanked the doctor for his clarification, explained the situation to Mr. Bentley (who was proud as a peacock to have "won" this battle with Attila the Nurse), and then informed Louise that she need not draw blood from Mr. Bentley. He was, in fact, going home. She felt a dull ache across her forehead as she finished solving yet another problem.

Then JoAnn remembered Flo and, for the second time, headed down the hall.

But she didn't get very far. Two rooms down the hall from Mr. Bentley's room, there was another argument going on. This time the problem was between Marion from Housekeeping and Ruth, one of the best nurses on the floor clinically, but one of the most stubborn people JoAnn had ever met.

To JoAnn's astonishment, the two women were debating the size of a spill beside a patient's bed. Ruth was insisting that the water on the floor constituted a "big spill," meaning it was Housekeeping's job to clean it up. Just as adamantly, Marion was insisting it was a "little spill," meaning it was the nurse's responsibility, not hers.

As JoAnn looked on, wondering what to do, the patient decided she'd heard enough. She picked up the pitcher of water on the table beside her bed and purposefully poured it on the floor.

"There," she said smugly. "Now we can all agree that this is a BIG spill. Will someone please clean it up so I can go back to bed and get the rest I need?"

JoAnn walked away, shaking her head in disbelief. "What next?" she wondered.

When JoAnn got to the nurses' lounge, Flo was nowhere to be found. One of the other nurses said she'd seen Flo going into the old research lab yesterday, so JoAnn decided to look there.

Upon entering the lab, JoAnn was astounded at the contraption she saw. There were boxes with lights and dials and a tangle of wires running everywhere.

"What's all this?" she grumbled.

She sat down in the only chair in the room and, in doing so, hit her elbow on the return key of the computer keyboard. There was a high-pitched whine, a blinding flash of light, and JoAnn Mode was transported to the 12th Dimension.

4

Of course, JoAnn did not know she was in the 12th Dimension. But she knew something had happened. Because, looking around, she saw things were different.

For instance, purple fog was drifting across the floor.

"This is not normal," thought JoAnn.

And little, crinkly lightning bolts were flitting here and there all around Flo's invention in the old research lab.

"No, this definitely is not normal," thought Jo-Ann.

And from the contraption to which all the wires ran, there came a strange pinkish glow.

"This is so *ab*normal, I'm leaving!" thought JoAnn.

So she backed away. JoAnn tiptoed through the purple fog, found the door, and stepped out into the hall, hoping that everything would be normal again. But everything was not. In fact, everything was even stranger.

The fog was thicker and multicolored. People were scurrying around, whirling and twirling in all directions, bouncing off one another, and tripping over huge stacks of papers.

As JoAnn was pondering the perplexity of it all, the hall became filled with a ghastly green light. From around the corner came a big, scaly troll. JoAnn began to back away as the troll stomped toward her. Then she noticed something remarkable. Its claws had fingernail polish.

Fire engine-red fingernail polish. Yes, it was exactly the shade always worn by . . .

JoAnn looked up into the face of the troll and saw that it was the face of her boss, Mary Ellen Krabofski! She was carrying printouts of some post-surgery data under one greenish arm, and she walked right past JoAnn without even seeing her.

Keeping her distance, JoAnn followed her boss through the fog as Mary Ellen headed straight for JoAnn's office—and straight up to a faint, ice-blue blur, which turned out to be the assistant nursing supervisor, Phyllis.

"Where's JoAnn Mode?" asked Mary Ellen, her tail twitching.

Phyllis, whose desk was surrounded by sandbags, dove for cover against the expected incoming barrage.

"She's out," muttered Phyllis.

"Well, when she gets back," said Mary Ellen, as one of the computer printouts she was holding curled up into a large, black ball and sprouted a smoldering fuse, "you give her this."

And she tossed the black ball over the sandbags to Phyllis. As Mary Ellen left, a pool of ghastly green followed her.

Phyllis quickly took the black ball and its sputtering fuse into JoAnn's office and dropped it on her desk.

JoAnn looked around. "Why is everyone moving so strangely?" she wondered. "Why is it so foggy? Where are the fluorescent lights?"

All the normal people were here. JoAnn saw them running around in the fog, though she did have a little trouble recognizing some of them.

The only person who didn't seem to be in fast-forward was good old Mrs. Estello, who looked like a dim ember sitting in the shadows. Mrs. Estello was in slow motion as she sat there in her normal unit clerk's chair, pecking away at a computer keyboard—mindlessly making error after error without a break.

"Excuse me," said JoAnn. "Aren't you going to correct those mistakes?"

But Mrs. Estello's fingers did not even pause.

Peeking into a room, JoAnn saw a mechanical woman standing beside a patient's bed. Looking closely, she could see it had the face of one of the surgeons, Dr. Clayton, who kept mumbling the same words over and over again—sounding just as monotonous as she always sounded talking with her patients. Her voice had no life. Her words had no warmth. She was a doctor who might as well have been a robot.

In another room, JoAnn saw Dr. Marcus jumping around like a kangaroo, while a wide-eyed patient looked on in astonishment. As Dr. Marcus hopped from one side of the patient's bed to the other, he bellowed out orders, using a large, rusty megaphone to be sure that no one missed a word. The attending nurse was shaking in her shoes, teeth rattling and voice quivering as she said repeatedly, "Y-y-yes, Dr. Marcus." The patient pulled the covers up over his head.

JoAnn turned to walk back toward the nurses' station, but she could hardly make her way because the dark fog kept visibility low. She found that she had to step over papers that were strewn throughout the hall. Big stacks, little stacks. To JoAnn, it seemed there were papers *everywhere*.

JoAnn quickly discovered that she wasn't the only one having trouble with the paper mess. Everywhere she looked, nurses were tripping and bumping into one another, trying to avoid the stacks of paper.

To JoAnn's surprise, she saw that when the nurses failed to step carefully, the papers stuck to their feet like glue. No matter how hard they tried to remove the sticky sheets from their shoes, they stayed stuck. Once they'd been joined together, it seemed to JoAnn there was just no separating the nurses from the papers.

As JoAnn neared the nurses' station, she could hear a strange noise. It came from a huge clock that was as large as the wall on which it hung. Its ticks and tocks were so loud that JoAnn had to cover her ears. The nurses in the station were struggling to concentrate on their reports when GONG!—another hour marked its passing. JoAnn watched as the nurses moved their pens even faster, trying to keep up with the quick pace of the mammoth clock's loud ticking.

Shaking her head in astonishment, JoAnn went back out into the hall. There, a whitish form came shuffling out of the fog, emerging as a woman wrapped in mummy tape. The mummy appeared to be Donna, one of JoAnn's Med-Surg nurses. She seemed to be tied up in administrative knots, as she normally was. Donna was one of those nurses who was usually so busy trying to deal with administrative issues—like creating new staffing charts—that she hardly ever had enough time to care for her patients.

"Hey, Donna," called JoAnn. "What's happened here?"

But Donna kept on shuffling by, passing JoAnn as she went about her work.

Wandering down the hall—and being very careful where she stepped—JoAnn was shocked to see some of her nurses and aides riding skateboards, carefully weaving in and out of the stacks of paper as they distributed meds and answered patients' calls.

Throughout the unit she observed obstacles set up in the form of barricades and wooden hurdles that seemed to have the sole purpose of making things difficult for everyone. People had to crawl over them, slowing their progress as they tried to respond to patients. JoAnn noticed that a few people were trying to squeeze by the barricades. Some made it, but others got stuck.

Just then, some hospital volunteers walked by. They were surrounded by a pale yellow fog. Their pace was uneven, and they didn't seem to have any clear direction about where they were going. They, too, tried to avoid getting stuck in the strewn papers or bumping into the racing, whirling nurses and aides.

What was wrong with everybody? JoAnn had never seen her unit like *this* before.

"What's happened to everybody? Why isn't anybody talking to me?!" cried JoAnn in frustration.

"Because they can't see or hear you," said a voice behind her.

JoAnn turned around to see Flo.

"Flo! What in the world is going on?" asked JoAnn. "Is this some kind of dream, nightmare, or what?"

"None of the above," Flo said. "We're both in the 12th Dimension."

And she and JoAnn sat down while Flo explained the Flo-Vision.

"Remember when I told you about my new invention?" Flo asked JoAnn.

"No," JoAnn replied. "I guess I wasn't really listening."

"Well," said Flo, "I was trying to tell you about the Flo-Vision. It's this great machine I've invented. I built it in the old research lab, with the help of someone I know in Biomedical Engineering. My friend and I like to tinker with things and, well, we did it! We created the Flo-Vision! It lets us look at our work areas and patient care in a way that nobody has ever been able to before."

"But why is everything so different here?" JoAnn asked.

"It isn't different," said Flo. "We're just seeing things we can't see in the normal world."

"Like what?"

"Like how people feel about what they're doing; what it's like for them on the *inside,*" said Flo.

"Come on! These can't be the people on *my* unit," said JoAnn. "This is ridiculous. Take me back to the real world."

Normally, Flo would have been intimidated by JoAnn Mode and would have kept her mouth shut. But here in the 12th Dimension, where she had discovered far more than her supervisor, she was bold enough to look JoAnn in the eye, shake her head, and say, "You just don't get it, do you?"

"Get what?"

"Look around. JoAnn, this *is* the real world," said Flo. "It's the same place, but we're seeing it in a different way. That's what the Flo-Vision is all about. Did you notice that most of the light around here comes from people?"

"Now that you mention it. . . ."

"Take Mrs. Estello. Her light is so dim that it doesn't even make it to her fingertips," said Flo. "On the other hand, Mary Ellen Krabofski has a lot more, but her light doesn't shine very far beyond herself, does it?"

"So?" asked JoAnn.

"I think we're seeing an invisible power that people have—invisible in the normal world, but visible in the 12th Dimension," said Flo.

"Well, that's very interesting," said JoAnn. "But let's get out of here and go back to work. If the rest of the 12th Dimension is this scary, then whatever you're talking about isn't worth bothering with."

"But every place isn't like this." said Flo. "Some are even worse!"

"Oh, terrific."

"But wait—some are *wonderful*! And there is one place you have to see before we go back. It's so bright there that, well, you'll just have to see it to believe it."

"Well, I'd love to, but . . ."

"Really, I insist," said Flo.

So JoAnn, realizing that Flo was pretty much in the driver's seat here, said, "OK, show me."

And they went off together through the multicolored fog and mist.

5

It seemed to JoAnn that they had journeyed a great distance, though, in fact, it had not been very far at all. As the mist thinned, they walked out of the pastel-colored fog into a brighter area.

"Where are we?" asked JoAnn.

"We're in the Radiology department," answered Flo.

The walls they saw here gave structure, but did not confine. And this place did not feel stationary; it felt as if it were in motion.

Most astounding, though, were the people, who emitted a mysterious light. Some were brighter than others, but their collective brilliance was like a small, warm sun.

The radiologists and technologists were busy, but they all moved about with purpose. There was less wasted energy and less confusion than Flo and JoAnn had seen in the other units at Normal Medical Center.

Suddenly Flo called out, "Look! There she is! Watch that woman over there!"

As she spoke, she pointed to a small, robust woman in a cone-shaped wizard hat who wandered about.

"Why is she so special?" asked JoAnn.

"You'll see," said Flo, knowingly.

Just then a door swung open, and a young knight staggered out. The suit of armor he wore was battered and scorched. His helmet plumes were burned to cinders. His sword was chipped and cracked. Through the door, Flo and JoAnn could see a dragon behind him, panting fire.

The woman in the wizard hat approached the knight. She was talking to him when, suddenly, right in front of them, a bolt of lightning appeared in her hand.

The bolt forked and flickered and flashed in the woman's hand.

Then, with a graceful windup, she pitched the lightning straight at the young man, as JoAnn and Flo ducked.

"*Zapp!*" went the lightning through the air. And right into the man.

JoAnn and Flo flinched, fearful that the young man would be dead on the floor. But, to the contrary, instantly he became more alive and glowed brightly.

One by one, the dents in his armor popped out. The scorch marks vanished. New plumes sprouted from his helmet as the charred cinders of the old plumes fell off. His sword became whole again. And he marched back to face the dragon once more.

The door to the room closed behind him. There were roars and shrieks, clangs of metal, blasts of fire, and all kinds of other noises.

The woman quietly moved on.

She walked down to the far end of the unit and looked out the window. Flo and JoAnn followed to see what it was outside that was so interesting. As they looked down on a square area surrounded by high walls, they could hardly believe their eyes.

The first thing they noticed was all the activity. Two radiologists, several technologists, and a few clerical employees were just finishing helping some patients move through what appeared to be a complicated outdoor maze made up of hedges over six feet tall. As they made their way through the winding maze, the patients and staff alike were being careful not to bump into the high, prickly hedges that lined the path on both sides.

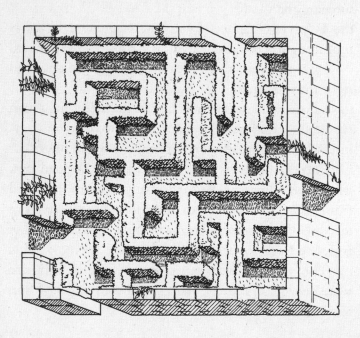

Because the radiologists and staff were familiar with the maze, they were able to guide the patients at every turn, moving as quickly as they could.

That's when it hit Flo that the grass didn't look normal.

"Look, JoAnn, the grass down there isn't really grass. It's *Astroturf*. Just like the artificial turf on a football field," said Flo.

"You're right," said JoAnn, still confused.

Flo and JoAnn turned to look at each other in utter amazement. *What was going on here?*

They glanced over at the woman in the wizard hat who was watching as the last patient was escorted through a small hole in the wall. And then, to their surprise, the wizard woman pointed her finger toward the group outside.

A huge, new bolt of lightning forked and flickered and flashed in the woman's hand. As the woman began to call to the people, *Zapp!* went the lightning, branching out to every person in the group. And each of them glowed brighter than before.

The woman left, but JoAnn and Flo stayed to watch the group as they huddled together to talk among themselves. Little flickers of lightning passed among them. Then the group broke up into two or three smaller groups. One group got out stop watches and tape measures to monitor how long it took to get from point to point. Another group got a tall ladder so that they could see the maze from up above. Others started to make a map.

"Well, I'll be . . ." said JoAnn.

"I thought you'd be impressed," glowed Flo.

"Say, Flo, who do you think these people are?"

"They're all part of the Radiology department," said Flo. "And they sure have their act together."

As they walked away from the window, they noticed a woman in the patient waiting area answering a phone call. Little by little, as she handled the call, she began to glow with lightning. After she hung up the phone, they saw her put two fingers to her lips and blow a shrill whistle.

With a clatter of hooves, a silver horse came prancing over to the woman. Suddenly the theme song from "The Lone Ranger" began to play. She gathered up some papers that were tied in a neat bundle, climbed up on the silver horse, and took the reins.

"Charge!" she yelled, and rode off, the music fading as it followed her down the hall.

Meanwhile, the noises coming from the dragon lair down the hall had slowly diminished. The door opened again. Out came the young man.

His armor was battered again, and his plumes were singed. But this time, the dragon followed him . . . meekly. On a leash. And everyone realized that he had not only fought the dragon, he had tamed it.

6

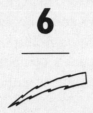

Both JoAnn Mode and Flo Knight were fascinated by this incredible sight of human lightning flashing among people and everyone working away at these amazing tasks.

Meanwhile, back in the real world, Mary Ellen Krabofski, fuming at the hospital's inability to hire good nurses these days, had gone to the Med–Surg unit to see JoAnn Mode. She was furiously searching the unit for JoAnn so that she could complain about the most recent patient report.

She stomped into the nurses' lounge and learned from some of the nurses that JoAnn had been seen going into the old research lab down at the end of the hall. So Mary Ellen trudged to the end of the hall and walked into the last room on the right. Immediately, she tripped over an extension cord, which yanked the plug out of the wall and sent her reeling headfirst into the Flo-Vision.

The Flo-Vision went dead, and Mary Ellen Krabofski went limp on the floor.

All of a sudden, JoAnn and Flo began to feel peculiar. For a few seconds they were not solid anymore. And, before their eyes, the lightning Zapping among everyone dissolved.

The young man's armor became a normal hospital uniform.

The dragon became a computer disk.

The wizard became a rather ordinary-looking woman.

The turf-covered field outside became just a plain table around which a group of people were laughing and talking.

JoAnn and Flo found that they had suddenly materialized in the middle of the Radiology department at Normal Medical Center. In a panic, they were looking for someplace to hide, when the rather ordinary-looking woman turned toward them. JoAnn recognized her immediately: It was Claire Burton, the radiology supervisor.

Surprised to see JoAnn and Flo bumping into each other as they attempted to get away unnoticed, Claire said, "Welcome to Radiology! May I help you with something?"

"No, thanks," said JoAnn sheepishly. "We're just walking around some of the other units in the hospital."

"Why didn't you say so?" asked Claire with a smile. "We've made some changes, and I'd like to show you how we've reorganized."

She led them around the department. The technologists they met along the way proudly explained the extra time they were spending with their patients and how well the patients seemed to like the new, streamlined procedures. Flo and JoAnn looked at each other, thinking the same thing: *Their* unit nurses didn't get this excited when they talked about changing the systems. And *extra* time? They never had *enough* time.

Although it looked like any other hospital unit, there was something different in the air. The radiologists and technologists here were so *involved* in what they were doing.

JoAnn and Flo could not see the lightning, but they could sense that it was there.

The radiologists and technologists worked as a coordinated team, helping one another whenever possible. They all seemed to know what to do—and how to do it effectively. They worked with purpose. They talked with purpose. There was a quiet hustle and bustle throughout the place.

"This is Tony," Claire said, pointing out a young man holding a computer disk. Flo and JoAnn noticed right away that this was the same man who, in the 12th Dimension, had worn the armor. Tony told them that he was the newest Radiology technologist at Normal Medical Center.

Then Claire said, "Tony found a *dragon* of a problem with the computer program that runs our film developer. He kept trying one thing after another to fix it. He thought it had him beat this afternoon, but we talked for a while and he went back and kept trying until he found the solution. We're all very proud of him."

Just then, the woman who had ridden off on the silver horse came through the door.

"Here comes Pam, one of our unit clerks," said Claire. "This morning she got a call from a doctor in Russia who was treating one of our former patients. The man became ill while he was there on vacation, and the Russian doctor needed some x-rays we took two years ago. Even though Pam had a lot of other work to do, she offered to find the x-rays and get them sent as soon as possible. When Pam found that the only available courier service was about to close out its last shipment for the day, she gathered up the films and rushed them to the courier service right away—and on her lunch hour, too."

They could almost hear "The Lone Ranger" theme playing again.

Then they went to a large room where two radiologists, some technologists, and a few clerical employees were talking and working together.

Not wanting to interrupt them, Claire spoke softly: "This is a team we put together to come up with ways to streamline the procedures here in Radiology. We want to be able to move patients in and out of our unit as quickly as possible. Some of our patients are quite sick, and some are uncomfortable waiting for long periods of time, so we're trying to shorten the *maze* of procedures that can get in the way of providing fast service."

"Hmm," thought JoAnn. "They're tackling everyday challenges. But it's more than routine; it has more meaning to them. It all seems so personally important to everyone on the team."

"You really have something special going on here in your department," Flo said to Claire.

"Well, we have a lean staff, but our patient satisfaction indices show that we are on the right track. We have been able to handle a 20 percent increase in volume this year without increasing our staff— just think of the money that saves the hospital. Everyone in the department seems happy, and the other departments tell us our service and quality have never been better," Claire explained. "I'd say we must be doing a few things right. I'm quite proud of our staff."

JoAnn noticed that she was beginning to feel more than a slight twinge of envy. What was it that made Claire's department so good? Did she have some kind of advantage nobody else had?

"You must have your choice of excellent personnel to do as well as you do," suggested JoAnn.

"No, I just work with the people I'm sent," said Claire.

"Then you must have more volunteers than everybody else," said JoAnn.

"Look around," laughed Claire. "We have the same number of volunteers as every other department."

"Different personnel policies?" asked JoAnn, getting desperate.

"I wish we did," said Claire. "But we have the same policies as everybody else in the hospital."

"Then what *are* you doing that makes this unit so good?" asked JoAnn.

"Well, it's only partly what *I* do. It's what we *all* do," she explained.

"I know what it is!" exclaimed Flo. "It's the lightning!"

For this outburst, Flo got JoAnn's elbow poked in her ribs.

"The *what*?" asked Claire incredulously.

"Nothing," said JoAnn. "She just means that everybody seems so *energized* around here."

"Oh," said Claire. "Well, I do think everyone feels good about being here. And I do my best to keep them charged up."

"And just how do you do that?" asked JoAnn, leaning forward.

"I'd like to think it's just being a good supervisor," she answered.

This reply definitely did not satisfy JoAnn, but by now they were at the door leading out of the Radiology department. Flo and JoAnn thanked Claire for her time, and headed back to the Med–Surg unit.

7

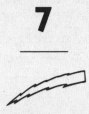

Med-Surg was operating normally when JoAnn and Flo returned to the nurses' station. Doctors, nurses, and aides were everywhere, and the conversations were normal.

"How much time before the shift ends?" someone was asking. "Another 10 minutes? I'll never make it!"

Someone else was saying, "I don't have time to finish these reports. Let the next shift worry about them."

And over in the corner, "We shouldn't have to straighten up the patients' rooms. We should complain to JoAnn about the Housekeeping staff not doing their jobs."

Still another was saying, "Where is the nursing supervisor? She's never around. She's always in meetings. I wish I had a job like that . . . always sitting around. I'd like to see her try to take care of all these patients. That's where the real work is."

Just then, all the nurses noticed that the boss was

back, and the whole place went silent. One by one, all the nurses and aides left the station.

At this point, however, JoAnn and Flo were feeling pretty good—especially Flo. Her invention was finished, and it had worked. She knew she had created something important—an entirely new way of looking at hospital work areas and patient care. She had shown it to her boss, and JoAnn seemed to be impressed.

"Things are going to work out fine," Flo thought to herself. And she headed for the old research lab to make sure the equipment was turned off.

But it was not to be that simple.

Back in the lab, Mary Ellen Krabofski was just getting up from the floor. Her yelling began the moment she laid eyes on Flo.

What was this stupid contraption she had stumbled into? Had senior management approved it? Did the unit's nursing supervisor know about it? If not, why wasn't she aware of it—after all, she was supposed to know *everything* about *everything*. What kind of a nursing supervisor was JoAnn Mode for allowing unauthorized projects in Med-Surg? Didn't Flo Knight know that extension cords were not allowed on the unit? Things certainly had not been like this when she had been a nurse.

"Send for JoAnn!" shouted Mary Ellen.

Gladly, Flo did this, so that someone else would have to deal with her.

JoAnn arrived, and Mary Ellen went on and on.

She even mentioned that workers' comp might have to pay for her hurt foot. In the end, Flo got the worst of it. She was forbidden to work on her crazy device ever again. In fact, she was ordered to dismantle it before she went home. She was to receive a letter of reprimand from Mary Ellen, and JoAnn was to watch Flo's every step.

Flo reluctantly did as she was told and started to dismantle her pride and joy.

JoAnn headed for her office, passing Mrs. Estello, who was on the phone saying, "Bandage order? How should I know? Oh, all right. I'll transfer you to someone else . . . oops!"

JoAnn looked at Mrs. Estello, and Mrs. Estello looked at JoAnn. It had been a long day for both of them.

"I guess we were disconnected," said Mrs. Estello. "Oh, well."

"*Nope, no lightning here*," thought JoAnn.

She went into her office and sat down at her desk. As soon as she looked at the printout from Mary Ellen, JoAnn felt as if it had exploded in her face. But the day had not been a total waste. Because JoAnn had seen lightning. Human lightning. She had seen the Zapp!

8

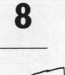

JoAnn Mode began to wonder.

Why, she wondered, if she was running her unit in the normal way, did her nurses and aides not have enough time to do all the things they knew were important? In the Radiology department, Claire's staff and the radiologists seemed to find enough time to do everything.

Why did she keep getting yelled at by Mary Ellen for not being good enough, while Claire was delivering great performance?

What was Claire Burton doing that she was not?

Well, whatever it was, Claire had the kind of commitment and morale JoAnn wanted in her unit.

Surely it had to do with the lightning bouncing back and forth among the Radiology department staff. What was that lightning? What made it work?

Then JoAnn realized, "Hmm, this could be it . . . the answer to my problems."

So she got out her notebook.

JoAnn Mode's Notebook

If I figure out what the lightning is, then:

- I can use it in my unit.
- Patients will receive better care and be happier.
- We can meet the quality and productivity goals senior management is always talking about.
- Nursing will be more fun.
- Maybe Mary Ellen will lighten up.
- Life will be simpler—and better.
- I could become an outstanding nursing supervisor.
- I might even get a raise!

"And if *she* can do it, *I* can do it!" thought JoAnn. But how?

Of course, the easy thing to do would have been to go to Claire, talk with her directly and openly, and try to learn from her.

"Nah!" JoAnn entertained that possibility for only a split second. That would have violated her Three Ironclad Rules:

1. Never ask for help.
2. Never let it seem that you can't handle everything on your own.
3. And never, ever talk to anyone about anything important unless you have no choice.

Besides, if she could do this on her own, she might be able to grab all the credit. So JoAnn decided she would figure it out by herself. The first thing she did was to give the lightning a name.

She called it Zapp!

JoAnn Mode's Notebook

Zapp! . . .

A force that energizes people.

Now, how could she generate Zapp! in the Med-Surg unit? The problem was that you couldn't see Zapp!, but you knew it was there. Kind of like excitement and enthusiasm. JoAnn remembered that in Radiology, everyone on the staff had seemed proud of what they were doing.

"Aha!" thought JoAnn. "Claire must give them pep talks. She must be a motivator."

So the next day, JoAnn called a brief staff meeting and tried giving a pep talk.

But nothing much happened. A few people seemed to be enthusiastic for about five minutes; then everyone went back to being the way they had been before.

JoAnn did some more thinking. "Let's see . . . Claire was nice to everybody," she thought. "So I'll try to be extra nice for a while."

But that didn't work either. Most people were nice in return, but nobody did a better job or became more committed to their work as a result.

"Well, that didn't work," thought JoAnn. "If being nice didn't make any lightning, then I'll be mean!"

But being mean turned out to be no more effective than being nice. Actually, it made things worse. Both the professional staff and the service personnel jumped when JoAnn appeared, only to slack off when she turned her back. Tensions ran high. Morale plummeted. Worst of all, patient care suffered.

Not only that, but after JoAnn did some checking around, she learned that it was extremely rare for Claire Burton to raise her voice to any of her staff. Yet all the Radiology employees applied themselves, got things done on time with outstanding results, and readily accepted responsibility.

What could she do next?

JoAnn thought, "Hey, I bet Zapp! is nothing more than one of those new programs the hospital is always promoting!"

She looked into it and, indeed, Radiology did have innovative programs. But then, Med-Surg—and other units—had programs, too.

So, it seemed to JoAnn, special programs were not the same as Zapp!

By now, JoAnn was stymied. So she decided to visit the hospital library. She came across a well-worn nursing journal on one of the dusty shelves. It mentioned something called "shared governance."

Whatever Happened to Shared Governance?

Shared governance stems from the idea of involving all hospital professionals in the decision-making process. The basic idea has been around for a long time, but it has had its ups and downs in terms of popularity. It has also been known by other names, like "participative management" and "employee involvement."

One of the big problems is that hardly anybody understands what it really means. Some nurse managers think it means being friendly to employees. Others think it means being sensitive to the needs and motivations of people. Still others think it means asking employees for help or having lots of group meetings.

Using it, different nurse managers get different results. One nurse manager calls a meeting and tries to get people involved—and it works. Another nurse manager does the same thing—and nothing happens.

While shared governance has not been a failure, confusion over what it is—and what it is not—has prevented widespread success.

Could the Radiology department be using shared governance? JoAnn wasn't sure. Med–Surg had tried programs in the past where they'd asked for nurses' ideas. Wasn't that shared governance? She was confused.

Then JoAnn read other articles about job satisfaction, job enrichment, and various other kinds of programs. But she was sure Radiology had none of these, or she would have heard about them at the regular monthly meetings for unit supervisors.

Maybe it had something to do with the way the Radiology department was organized.

The entire hospital had gone through a reorganization last year that had involved the removal of some of the management personnel. In the hospital newsletter, the C.E.O. had called it a "flattened" staff organization. According to the C.E.O., reorganization was supposed to be a good thing. But everyone in the hospital knew that the real reason it had happened was because of the emphasis on reducing costs.

All JoAnn knew was that soon after the flattening process began, *she* nearly had been flattened by the weight of new responsibilities dropped on her, and she had almost lost her assistant nursing supervisor. It appeared to JoAnn that if there were good things about a flattened organization, only Radiology seemed to know about them.

Then JoAnn considered things like staff development, effective communication, closer supervisor-staff relationships, advanced training for technologists, and lots of other ideas.

In every case, if Radiology had them, they worked. If the other units had them, they didn't seem to matter much.

Now JoAnn was really stumped. Nearly all the ideas she'd considered were, she had to admit, very good ones. So she made a list.

JoAnn Mode's Notebook

Normal Medical Center units have tried:

- Staff development programs.
- Better communication.
- Closer supervisor-staff relationships.
- More interaction between doctors and nurses.
- Quality circles.
- Improved quality-of-work-life programs.
- New computer programs.
- Patient relations.
- Staff representatives at Board of Directors meetings.
- Hospital-community committees.
- Partnerships with businesses.
- Employment of consultants.
- Community resource people.
- And lots of other programs.

Notebook ▦ (cont'd)

What happened?

- Results were usually mixed, short lived, disappointing, counter-productive, confusing, or insignificant—in most of the hospital.
- They work well only when Radiology tries them.

Now what did that mean?

"That Radiology has the *key* to making all these other ideas and programs work, something we're still missing!" JoAnn concluded.

"That must be the lightning," thought JoAnn. "Whatever that Zapp! is, it must be powerful stuff."

She continued writing in her notebook.

JoAnn Mode's Notebook

Zapp! . . .

A key to success for new ideas and programs.

They work with Zapp!

They fail without Zapp!

But at this point, JoAnn saw that she was still no closer to understanding what Zapp! was. She knew that she needed help. So she decided to violate Ironclad Rule Number One.

9

By now, Flo Knight was back to her normal routine. And because of the letter of reprimand, she really hated going to work every day.

The nurses' union, of course, had filed a grievance on her behalf, but that was an endless bureaucratic voyage, and Flo wasn't sure she wanted to go that route. Right now, she just wanted to be left alone by everyone, especially Mary Ellen Krabofski and JoAnn Mode.

Meanwhile, Flo's attitude was consistently negative. She took care of her patients, and she filled out the required reports. But there was no spring in her step. She felt as if her spring had sprung.

This was not a good time to talk to Flo about much of anything that had to do with work.

But JoAnn Mode knew that she needed help, and that Flo was the only one in the hospital who would understand what she was talking about.

So she went to Flo one day near the end of their shift.

"Look, Flo, I want to figure out what that lightning was in Claire Burton's unit. I can't do it on my own, and I was wondering if you'd help me."

"You want *me* to help *you*? Forget it!" shouted Flo.

"OK," said JoAnn. "I admit you got a bad break. But if you'll help me out on this, I'll submit your invention to senior management for approval."

"Take it to senior management? Ha!" said Flo. "Don't make me laugh! They won't do anything except remind me that I'm a nurse, not an inventor."

"But think about it," encouraged JoAnn. "To help me, you'll have to reassemble the Flo-Vision. You can start using it again, and it'll be with my blessing. That way, I'll take the blame if Mary Ellen Krabofski is unhappy."

"Well . . ." said Flo.

"And if we can figure out what the lightning is and what makes it go *Zapp!*, then we can use it here on our unit, and you'll have been a part of that."

"Well . . ." said Flo.

"And later on, I'll even try to get you some time in your schedule so you can keep developing your invention. You said you thought this was important, that it could help us make the unit a better place for our patients. What do you say? Are we going to work together on this?"

"Well . . ." said Flo. "OK!"

They shook hands, both genuinely excited. Had they observed what was going on from the 12th Dimension, they would have seen a very small bolt of lightning flash between them.

10

Flo hurried to work the next morning with new interest and vitality, arriving an hour before the start of her shift. She even whistled as she left her car, heading toward the Normal Medical Center entrance. She was happy for a change. "Maybe I *can* make a difference," she thought.

She headed straight for the old research lab because she had a task to complete: the Flo-Vision.

Once in the lab, Flo quickly reassembled the Flo-Vision, fired it up, and vanished into the 12th Dimension.

As she wandered around the Medical-Surgical unit, the situation was still normal. Things were the same: papers sticking to everyone's feet as they hurried between patients, nurses and aides leaping high hurdles, the loud ticking of the unit clock ever present in the background.

In the midst of all this was JoAnn Mode, dressed that day (to the eyes of those in the 12th Dimension) in a cowboy hat, boots, and spurs. She looked like Annie Oakley, except she was toting a six-gun, ready to blast anyone who got in her way.

Flo was about to walk over to Radiology when she saw something she hadn't noticed before.

Flo watched as JoAnn walked up to Donna, the nurse who was wrapped in mummy tape. Soon after JoAnn started talking, there was a flash of—well, it was not lightning.

Instead of a flash of light, there was a flash of darkness.

Kind of like blinking your eyes.

And there was a sound.

It did not go *Zapp!*

It went *"Ssssappi"*

To Flo, it sounded like a balloon deflating. After the Sappi happened, Flo watched as a couple of more turns of mummy tape wound around Donna, making the light inside her a shade dimmer.

Then Flo noticed a member of the Housekeeping staff trying to say something to JoAnn. JoAnn walked away, not paying any attention to her.

Sappi

About that time, one of the unit's veteran nurses entered the office. She had just received an invitation to speak at a Career Day at a local high school, and she wanted to tell her boss the good news. But JoAnn didn't have time to listen. She said only, "That's nice," as she turned and walked away. The nurse left the office with her head lowered.

Sapp¡

Next, Flo heard JoAnn tell Phyllis how to do a job she had done many times before, without bothering to listen to how *she* thought it should be done.

Sapp¡

Flo then saw JoAnn rush over to an aide who was having a problem, immediately pull her off the job, and start solving the problem herself.

Sapp¡

But it wasn't just what JoAnn was doing. It was also what she was *not* doing. Flo heard some of the nurses complaining that they had no idea how well they were doing their jobs. "JoAnn was supposed to evaluate all of us last month," explained Sam. "But then she didn't—she said she had other, more important things to do."

Sapp¡

The nurses were even doing it to each other. She heard one nurse telling some others, "That's not our problem. Let the nursing supervisor worry about it."

Sapp¡

The doctors were doing it to the nurses, too. One doctor was saying to a nurse, "I've explained this to you a dozen times before! Don't you ever listen?"

Sapp¡

And the doctors and nurses could be heard blaming

the other departments for taking too long with test results. One nurse was telling a doctor, "It isn't *our* fault! The other departments are always late, and then *we* have to deal with the patients' complaints. How can we do our jobs when the other units are so slow?!"

Sapp¡

Worst of all were the comments some of the nurses were making to patients.

"Mr. Gary, there really is nothing I can do. It is the hospital's policy."

Sapp¡

"Please, Mrs. Jackson, I have many other patients. I'm doing the best I can."

Sapp¡

"What's going on here?" Flo wondered. These were routine, everyday, *normal* occurrences—nothing that most people would notice.

But whenever these things happened, people got dimmer. Some slowed down, doing only what was absolutely necessary. Others kept up their pace but became more frantic and disorganized, getting less and less done.

Sometimes a few new stones would appear on the many walls crisscrossing the unit. There were more and more communication problems among the doctors, nurses, support staff, and aides, which kept them from providing the best patient care possible. It also kept them from making much progress toward their cost-control goals. Whatever was happening, it was draining their energy or damming it up so it couldn't be used.

And JoAnn Mode was a big part of it. She went through the day Sapping people left and right. And in the same way she Sapped her nurses and aides, they Sapped their patients.

"She's like a black hole, absorbing energy from everyone who works for her," thought Flo, as she returned to the normal world and started her shift.

At the end of the shift, Flo decided to visit the 12th Dimension. She saw that the majority of the Med–Surg nurses and aides were frazzled and de-energized. When the clock showed that it was quitting time, everyone headed for the exit, glad the day was over.

Flo watched them go, rushing for the fix of energy they needed from home, family, friends, and the things they did *after* work. She wandered back through the multicolored fog toward JoAnn's office. When she got there, she saw that her supervisor was in trouble.

JoAnn was alone in the midst of an enormous cloud of flashing darkness. She was beaten and bruised, standing her ground as jaws and claws came out of the fog and mist from all directions. She had been bravely firing away with her six-gun but there were many monsters and her gun was now empty.

What was this thing confronting JoAnn? Flo stood and watched her fight her losing battle. And then Flo had a hunch what it was.

It was everything JoAnn had Sapped from everyone else. What JoAnn had taken away, had not shared, was now beating her. What was it?

It was Responsibility.

It was Authority.

It was Accountability.

It was Challenge.

It was Recognition.

It was Trust.

11

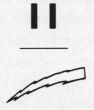

Of course, JoAnn Mode did not believe any of this stuff about Sapp¡ and the cowboy hat and the six-gun.

"Then go take a look for yourself," Flo challenged. "It's not just in our unit. It's everywhere in the hospital."

JoAnn walked down the familiar hall to the old research lab. After entering the proper commands on the Flo-Vision, she found herself in the 12th Dimension. Invisible to the normal world, JoAnn walked around her unit.

She saw a doctor who was supposed to be leading a discussion group. But there was no discussion. The doctor was doing all the talking. Even when the doctor asked a question, she jumped in and told the nurses the answer. The doctor seemed to enjoy hearing herself talk, but the nurses were getting more and more frustrated by the minute.

Sapp¡

She saw a nurse taking all the credit for an idea a *team* of nurses had come up with.

Sapp¡

Down the hall, JoAnn saw several nurses and aides gathered around the unit's bulletin board. They were reading the latest memo from the director of nursing. It said, "Henceforth, all hospital employees will punch time clocks when you arrive and when you leave. For every minute you arrive late, and for every minute you leave early, you will be docked 15 minutes of pay. This new policy is effective immediately."

Sapp¡

JoAnn went into the patients' lounge and found an L.P.N. talking with a patient's husband who was very angry. Tiny beads of sweat were breaking out on the nurse's forehead because the husband's complaint was related to a billing problem, not patient care. JoAnn had told the man to talk with someone else on the unit because she didn't want to handle any more problems that shift, and the Billing department was closed for the day. The nurse, who realized she had no authority to comment on a billing policy, just had to stand there and take it.

Sapp¡

Coming up the stairwell were two Med-Surg nurses who were upset because of the new mandatory training schedule JoAnn had posted yesterday. One of them said, "I had an important family trip that will have to be cancelled because of the new schedule. JoAnn Mode didn't check with any of us to see if the new schedule would be convenient."

The other nurse nodded her head. "That's normal," she said.

Sapp¡¡

JoAnn walked over to the nurses' station. She saw three aides discussing their adjusted work schedules.

"Every time the schedule is changed, it's a big hassle for all of us," one aide complained.

"Well," sighed one of the other aides, "there's not much we can do if the supervisor won't listen."

"These problems occur every couple of months," complained the third aide. "It seems nobody on this unit cares about our schedules except us."

"Let's do the best we can for a while until we can talk with the supervisor. I'll try to pin her down to a meeting, but she probably won't have time for us."

As the aides walked away, one of them said, "That's normal. She never has time to listen."

"What's the use?" another added.

Sapp¡¡¡

JoAnn continued her tour. Overall, she saw lots of Sapping and not very much Zapping going on.

When JoAnn came back to the normal world, she sat down with Flo and told her what she'd seen in the 12th Dimension. Together, they created quite a list of what Sapps people.

JoAnn Mode's Notebook

Examples of what Sapps people:

• Not being able to do everything you could do for patients.

• Lack of responsibility.

• Someone else solving problems for you.

• Assignments that are always the same.

• No way of determining how well others think you're doing.

• No way of measuring your own performance.

• No challenge.

• No authority.

• No time to solve problems.

• Not being listened to.

• Not getting credit for your ideas or efforts.

Notebook (cont'd)

- Believing that you can't make a difference.
- Rigid, bureaucratic policies.
- Confusion.
- Not enough knowledge or skills to do the job.
- Lack of support, coaching, and feedback.
- Poor communication.
- Not enough resources to do the job well.
- People treated exactly the same, like interchangeable parts.
- Lack of trust.

"Look," JoAnn said, after scanning the list. "Don't a lot of these examples have something in common?"

"Most of them have to do with confidence and trust—or, rather, the lack of them," said Flo.

"And self-esteem and control," said JoAnn.

"If the lack of these things Sapps people," said Flo, "I wonder what more confidence and trust, higher self-esteem, and less control would do?"

They looked at each other. Had they found the secret?

It was about then that JoAnn and Flo began to realize that Sapp¡ and Zapp! were halves of the same idea.

JoAnn Mode's Notebook

Zapp!—the giving of power?

Sapp¡—the taking of power?

12

Flo spent the next day invisibly observing Radiology and Med-Surg from the 12th Dimension. She wanted to learn more about how people feel when they are Zapped and Sapped. It didn't take long to notice some big differences between the Radiology department and the Medical-Surgical unit.

In Radiology, the technologists pretty much controlled their own jobs. They could make a lot of decisions on their own.

In Med-Surg, everybody had to check with JoAnn before doing anything.

The staff in Radiology acted as if their jobs were important to them and they were important to their jobs.

The staff in Med-Surg acted as if their jobs didn't much matter in the scheme of things, as long as the patients got what they needed.

Whether things went right or wrong, the technologists took it a bit personally in Radiology.

It was hard to know if things were going right or

wrong in Med–Surg. No matter how things went, though, the nurses and aides thought it was bad to take things personally or to get personally involved in making changes.

The staff in Radiology was so involved with their patients that they talked with each other about new equipment and improving their processes—sometimes even after work.

The staff in Med–Surg would look at you oddly if you said anything about trying to improve processes. The only acceptable topics during casual conversations were family matters, vacations, sports, and hobbies.

In Claire Burton's unit, the staff usually finished their work by the end of the shift. Even when they stayed later to finish the day's tasks, each employee left with a sense of accomplishment—tired, but still energized—and *wanting* to come back tomorrow.

In JoAnn Mode's unit, no one ever seemed to finish. Some employees hurried out when the shift ended, counting the days left to the next day off, retirement, or both. The rest stayed until they found a stopping place, frustrated and resentful. They never seemed to get anywhere and often dreaded coming back.

After a while in the 12th Dimension, Flo began to get an idea of how health care providers felt when they were Sapped and when they were Zapped. When she left the 12th Dimension, she hurried to talk with JoAnn. They entered their new insights into JoAnn's notebook.

JoAnn Mode's Notebook

When you have been *Sapped*, you feel like:

- Your job belongs to the hospital.
- You are just taking orders.
- You always have to keep your mouth shut.
- Your job is to *do*—not to come up with ideas about how to do things better or faster.
- Your job doesn't really matter.
- You don't know how well you're doing.
- You have little or no control over your work or patient care.
- Your job is different from who you are.
- You have to work harder because you aren't allowed to work smarter.
- You don't really matter.

Notebook 📖 (cont'd)

When you have been *Zapped*, you
feel like:

- Your job belongs to you.
- You are responsible.
- You have some say in how things
  are done.
- Your ideas are sought and valued.
- Your job counts for something.
- You know where you stand.
- You have some control over your
  work.
- Your job is a part of who you are.
- You're encouraged to work smarter,
  not harder.
- You know you really matter.

After much discussion, JoAnn and Flo came up
with some examples of what Zapps people. As they
talked, JoAnn scribbled in her notebook.

"We figured out what Sapps people. Now I think
we know what Zapps people," said JoAnn.

JoAnn Mode's Notebook

Examples of what Zapps people:

- Being able to use all your professional skills to help patients.
- Responsibility.
- Solving problems as a team.
- Variety in assignments.
- Measurable outputs.
- Ability to measure your own performance.
- Challenge.
- Authority to commit yourself and make decisions.
- Having the time to solve problems.
- Being listened to.
- Praise.

Notebook 📓 (cont'd)

- Recognition for ideas.
- Knowing why you're important to the system.
- Flexible controls.
- Direction (knowing what's important and how much or what quality is wanted).
- Knowledge and skills to do the job (training, staff development, continuing education, relevant information).
- Support, coaching, and feedback.
- Effective communication in all directions.
- Resources readily available.
- People treated like individuals, not like interchangeable parts.
- Trust.

They were definitely discovering something important, and they were pleased. Yet they wondered what they could *do* with their discoveries.

PART II

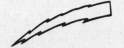

Zapping the Unit

13

JoAnn was excited about what she and Flo had found out. She was thinking about how she could create more Zapp! in the Med–Surg unit, when her phone began to ring.

"Hi, it's me," said Flo, when JoAnn answered.

"I was just about to come see you," said JoAnn.

"Well, here I am. I'm standing next to you in your office in the 12th Dimension, only you can't see me."

"Then how are you talking to me?"

"With my new cellular Flo-phone—the only telephone that works in the 12th Dimension," said Flo. "I invented a new backpack model so that I wouldn't have to keep going back to the normal world to talk to you."

"That's great," said JoAnn who, as usual, had no time for chitchat. "I have figured it out. It's simple. Zapped people own their jobs, they're responsible, they make decisions on their own—right? So I'll have everybody here be like that."

"But how?" asked Flo.

"Easy," said JoAnn. "I'll just call a staff meeting and tell them that's the way it's going to be."

JoAnn immediately asked the unit clerk to let everyone know that there would be a very short, special meeting near the end of the shift. JoAnn was quite proud of herself and spent the next hour thinking about how easy it would be to change the way things were in Med-Surg.

Ten minutes before the end of the shift, JoAnn hurried to the nurses' lounge to face a tired and confused staff.

JoAnn quickly called the meeting to order. Then, with a smile, she said, "I have great news for all of you. Things are going to change here in Med-Surg. So listen up, everybody. From now on, you own your jobs. They're all yours. I'm not making any decisions for you. Each of you can decide how you want to get your work done. You're in control. From this moment forward, I have complete confidence in all of you. Oh, by the way, your jobs are important, so start acting like it. And make sure all the doctors and patients are happy. Any questions?"

Of course, there were no questions because nobody understood what in the world she was talking about.

"Good. Everyone have a nice evening," said JoAnn.

Having made her speech, JoAnn returned to her office, put her feet up on her desk, and daydreamed fantasies of Mary Ellen Krabofski's congratulations for her great idea.

A few minutes later, Flo stopped by JoAnn's office. "JoAnn, I hate to tell you this, but I don't think things will go very well tomorrow. You confused and upset everyone at the meeting."

"What? Wasn't everybody Zapped after my speech?" asked JoAnn.

"I guess we'll see tomorrow morning."

And indeed, Flo was right. As soon as the shift started the next morning, Med-Surg was not normal. In fact, it was in a state of chaos.

One nurse decided she'd prefer to work a different shift the next day, but didn't coordinate her revised schedule with anyone else, leaving her scheduled shift shorthanded. Another nurse, who detested writing reports, elected not to write any reports at all the next day, telling her coworkers that "somebody else will just have to do it." All the aides got together and decided they would skip their lunch break so they could leave work an hour earlier than usual, which meant there were no aides on duty for the last hour of the shift. And Mrs. Estello decided that she was tired of dealing with problems from other departments, so she took her phone off the hook.

All around the unit, arguments were breaking out among the staff. They all wanted to do things *their* way.

Many people, though, were carrying on exactly as before, as if JoAnn's proclamation had never been made. After spending all their working lives in a state of Sappi, they didn't know what else to do.

JoAnn hurriedly got her staff together for another short meeting—something that was not normal for Med-Surg. She told everyone just to be normal, although she wasn't quite sure what that meant. "Remember what I said yesterday? Well, forget it. From now on, I'm in charge again. OK, go back to work."

Now everyone was doubly Sapped.

The whole matter was trickier than JoAnn Mode had figured. She retreated to her office with yet another headache and made an entry in her notebook.

JoAnn Mode's Notebook

It is easy to Sapp¡

It is hard to Zapp!

"Now what do I do?!" she asked aloud as she paced back and forth. "If I can't *talk* people into being Zapped, how can I make it happen?"

A moment later the phone rang. It was Flo, who had just entered the 12th Dimension. She was in JoAnn's office and could hear everything JoAnn was saying.

"You know, JoAnn, I've never seen Claire try to *talk* people into being Zapped. I don't think that's how she does it."

"Then what does she do?" asked JoAnn.

"Well . . ." said Flo. "I'm not sure exactly."

"OK, we're going to figure this out one way or another," said JoAnn. "Go to the Radiology department, find Claire, and shadow her. Find out *exactly* what she does. I'll cover for you here on the unit."

So Flo went off to check out the Radiology department.

An hour later, JoAnn's phone rang again. It was Flo with her first observation to report.

Flo had been watching Claire and noticed that whenever she talked to someone, she didn't put the person down or make the person feel inferior. Even if there was a problem, she said what she had to say so that people still felt, if not great, at least OK about themselves. That is, she always *maintained or enhanced the person's self-esteem*.

"OK, I'll try that out," said JoAnn. "You follow me now and watch what happens."

JoAnn thought for a moment and then went out into the hallway. The first person she came to was Helena, a long-time nurse in Med-Surg.

"Helena, you're a very neat dresser," said JoAnn. "I especially like the way your shoes are always polished and how your uniforms are always crisp and fresh."

Then JoAnn saw Carol, another nurse, and said, "Carol, I really like the color of your new car. I saw it in the parking lot yesterday."

To this, Carol said, "Gee, thanks, JoAnn."

"But you know, Carol, you screwed up royally in how you handled that patient's complaint yesterday. I had to spend an hour getting him settled down. I suggest you shape up and never let it happen again."

Then JoAnn went back to her office and waited for Flo to call and tell her how she did.

"When you talked to Helena, nothing happened. No lightning, no Zapp!, nothing," said Flo. "And when you talked to Carol, you actually Sapped her."

"Why? I said nice things to both of them. Didn't that do anything for their self-esteem?"

"But JoAnn, you didn't say anything positive about their *nursing*. Claire doesn't go out of her way just to tell people they look nice or that she likes the cars they buy. She talks about things they're doing on the job. And remember, she never puts people down, even if there is a problem."

"OK," said JoAnn. "Let me try again."

She went back out again, found Helena, and said, "Helena, I like how your reports are always on time. You're very well organized, and I'm sure that helps you be a good nurse. Keep it up."

Then she found Carol and said, "Carol, what I was trying to say earlier was that I think you're usually a first-rate nurse. What happened yesterday was a mistake, but I hope you'll keep handling family complaints the way you usually do."

Carol nodded and said, "I'll try not to let it happen again."

"OK," said JoAnn. "You're a good nurse, and that's all I can ask."

A while later, JoAnn saw Shelby, one of the newest nurses in Med-Surg. "You showed good judgment in calling me this morning about Mrs. Carr, the patient in Room 317. She was in a lot of pain, and I'm glad she didn't have to wait until our regular rounds to get some relief."

After each of these conversations, Flo saw little flickers of lightning. They were small, barely visible, but they were there. She called JoAnn.

"Bingo!" said Flo. "You did it! You Zapped 'em!"

A few days passed, and JoAnn kept using words that would maintain or enhance her staff's self-esteem when she talked to them about their work.

In fact, she tried to say something constructive to each person on the unit every day. After all those years of being Sapped, she reasoned, it was going to take a lot of little Zapps to build up a positive charge in Med–Surg.

JoAnn was very careful with what she said because she was determined to Zapp! as many Med–Surg nurses and aides as possible. She figured that when her staff felt capable, responsible, and valued, then they would encourage these same qualities in others.

Flo was especially glad to see that the Zapps were starting to filter down to the patients. On one occasion, after JoAnn had complimented Nan, an aide, about how well she had handled a patient's adjustment to a new roommate, Nan turned to the patient, smiled, and then complimented him on his help with the situation.

The same day Flo watched as another aide told a

patient, "You look terrific, Miss Austen. You certainly don't look like someone who just had surgery!"

Shortly after JoAnn told one nurse how pleased she was with the individual care the nurse was giving a long-term patient, the nurse said to the patient, "Your leg is healing well, Mrs. Jackson. Your use of the information we reviewed to help you care for your leg is making a difference. And it shows!"

Flo saw a nurse walk over to a patient's mother, who had been visiting all day. Usually a very pleasant woman, the mother looked especially tired. Realizing that the mother was having trouble leaving, the nurse put her arm around the woman and said, "Don't worry. We'll give her the care she needs. If you can't rest or are worried, feel free to call us." The woman smiled.

"Was Zapp! contagious?" wondered Flo.

Flo soon discovered that the *quality* of what JoAnn said was important, too. People could tell when something she said was insincere or undeserved. In those cases, the Zapp! quickly turned into a Sapp¡

As time went by, Flo saw the little flickers of lightning in Med–Surg grow brighter, but they were small; nothing like the brilliance or size of the Zapps in the Radiology department.

Still, JoAnn felt good about what she had accomplished so far. As the shift ended, she thought for a minute and then pulled her notebook from her desk drawer.

JoAnn Mode's Notebook

1st principle of Zapp!:

**Maintain or Enhance
Self-esteem**

14

One morning a few weeks later, JoAnn and Flo both arrived at the hospital early, eager to learn more about this fascinating Zapp! stuff. They both wanted to find out how Med-Surg could glow even more brightly.

JoAnn said to Flo, "You did a good job last month observing what Claire was doing. I know we're on the right track. But enhancing self-esteem must be only the first step. Why don't you keep looking and see what else Claire does?"

Flo was only too happy to head back to the 12th Dimension. So as soon as she had arranged for JoAnn to cover for her, she pushed the appropriate Flo-Vision commands and headed for the Radiology department.

As Flo expected, amazing things were going on as usual. Monsters were being tamed, strange and wonderful structures and machines were being created, and new paths in the maze were being discovered. And the incredible lightning energizing all of this was Zapping brilliantly from Claire to her technologists and from the technologists to their patients.

Then Flo noticed something she thought was rather odd. While some of the lightning flashed when Claire talked, often she would just be there with someone, seemingly doing nothing, and Zapp!—a little bolt of lightning would jump from her to the next person. It was as if Claire could generate a Zapp! just by standing next to someone.

By now, Flo knew that Zapp! did not happen by itself. Claire had to be doing *something*. So she watched her some more.

Then she noticed that Claire was letting her technologists do the talking. She would be standing nearby, eyes focused on the other person, sometimes her head angled to one side. And as she did this, a little Zapp! would pass between her and the person talking.

What was she doing? Flo wondered.

Why, of course! She was **listening!**

She got on the Flo-phone, dialed JoAnn Mode, and told her excitedly, "Listening to people is another way to Zapp! them."

"So what's the big deal about that?" asked JoAnn. "I listen to people all the time."

Flo did not answer.

"Don't I listen to people?" asked JoAnn.

Still Flo said nothing.

"WELL, DON'T I?"

"Lots of times I'm not sure, JoAnn," said Flo.

"And why not?"

"Because you're doing other things while I'm talking, or you don't let me finish what I have to say, or you change the subject when I do finish," said Flo.

JoAnn took this in. Then she said, "OK, but how do you know *she's* really listening?"

"Well, because she's looking at the person, and she's nodding her head as if she understands."

"Oh, what the heck, Flo. My kids do that! And I never know if they're listening or not," said JoAnn.

"Wait a minute, I know," said Flo, remembering something that made the lightning glow brighter. "When the other person was finished talking, she repeated a little summary of what had been said."

"*So she really is listening*," thought JoAnn.

"All right, let me try it," she said to Flo.

And she did.

As soon as JoAnn stepped out of her office, Phyllis came over to her and started to talk about a problem she was having with a dietician.

JoAnn stood in front of her.

She looked her in the eye.

She focused her full attention on her.

She nodded her head as Phyllis made a point.

But after a few seconds, she found that it was hard to listen well. Even though Phyllis got to the point quickly, JoAnn's own thoughts kept coming faster than the words. JoAnn's thoughts seemed to cover up what she was hearing. If she didn't push her own thoughts aside and concentrate on Phyllis's words, she soon would not hear what Phyllis was saying.

When Phyllis was finished, JoAnn tried to summarize what Phyllis had said to let her know her boss had listened. But JoAnn found she had caught only the first part of what Phyllis had said.

Still, she tried it some more. That was another thing to JoAnn Mode's credit: She would always keep trying.

As she went through the unit, she practiced listening to people the rest of the day. And the next day. And the day after that.

After a while, JoAnn became pretty good at listening to people. Instead of letting her own thoughts clutter up the message she was hearing, she kept her mind busy with keeping a mental list of each point the person made. Then it was easy to give back a short summary. If she got a point wrong, the person to whom she had been listening could make the point clear.

JoAnn noticed something else important: Aside from letting people know she was paying attention to what they said, she also began to understand what was really going on in the unit.

Meanwhile, during her lunch hour each day, Flo used the Flo-Vision to see how JoAnn was doing.

As you might imagine, Flo was getting a big kick

out of checking up on her boss. At first, Flo wondered if JoAnn Mode would *ever* really listen to anybody. She even thought she might have the grim pleasure of telling JoAnn that the Zapps were not happening, that JoAnn would never learn.

But Flo was wrong.

In fact, to her surprise, JoAnn was doing quite well. Just by building self-esteem and by listening to people, the Sapps had become far fewer and the Zapps far more common. There was a weak but definite glow now around the nurses, the aides, and the patients in Med-Surg.

What really came as a surprise was that Flo did not even have to be in the 12th Dimension to notice it. She noticed that there was less tension on the unit. Problems seemed to get sorted out a little faster. People were starting to make suggestions. The staff and the patients seemed happier.

And yet, she did have to report that the Zapps JoAnn gave by listening were not of the magnitude Claire Burton gave. When JoAnn listened, the Zapp! would start to grow and glow as Claire's did. But then JoAnn would walk away, and the Zapp! would vanish. Sometimes it even became a Sapp¡

One day Flo was having trouble with a new feature of the Flo-Vision. So she told JoAnn about it.

"I stayed late yesterday to work on this problem. In fact, I was here all evening. But I just don't have the tools to make it work," explained Flo, sounding extremely frustrated.

JoAnn listened dutifully, nodded her head, and even repeated an accurate summary of what Flo had said.

Then JoAnn pivoted and walked away.

"Hey, JoAnn, wait a minute," Flo said.

JoAnn walked back and said, "What?"

"Is that all you're going to do?" asked Flo.

"What else do you expect?" asked JoAnn.

"At least some kind of response," said Flo.

JoAnn was puzzled. Hadn't she done the Zapping thing right? Hadn't she listened?

Suddenly Flo understood why JoAnn was not generating the maximum charge when she listened.

"JoAnn, I think there are two parts to this listening thing," said Flo. "The first part is listening. The second part is responding. You've got the listening part fine, but often you don't respond."

"OK," said JoAnn. "How about if I say, 'I heard you. Now get back to work.' "

"That makes me feel as if you just want to get rid of me," said Flo. "It's a Sapp¡"

"But I wasn't trying to get rid of you," said JoAnn. "In fact, I was going to try to get you the tools you need."

"Then why didn't you tell me that?" asked Flo.

To which JoAnn said, "All right then, how about

if I say, 'I heard what you said. I'll get you the necessary tools.' "

Flo considered this. "Well, that's better, but somehow it feels as if there is still something missing. I mean, I spent my entire evening working on this problem, and you didn't even acknowledge that."

Then JoAnn Mode suddenly got it. She had listened and responded to the words Flo had said, but not to the *tone* in which Flo had said them.

"OK, *I can tell you're very frustrated,* and I know that you are giving this project your all—even staying late to work on it in the evening," said JoAnn. "Why don't you concentrate on your normal responsibilities today, and I'll get you the tools you need."

When she said that, there was a big Zapp!, one that lasted longer and glowed brighter than before. JoAnn knew from that point on that she not only had to listen, she also had to **respond with empathy.**

From then on, after JoAnn listened to someone, she tried to give the person an appropriate answer by responding to more than just the actual, factual words. She was beginning to respond to the *feelings* behind the words.

This meant that JoAnn had to pay close attention to the context of what was being said, and take into account not only the person's tone of voice, but things like body language, facial expressions, and events leading up to the discussion.

When someone came to her with a problem, JoAnn often said something like, "OK, I understand you're upset. Let's try to work something out."

For instance, one day Flo watched as JoAnn talked with Carol. "I can understand that you're frustrated," began JoAnn. "I'd be upset, too, if I had to wait so long for a prescription from Pharmacy. Let me check with them to see how much longer it's going to be."

When approached with a request from one of her staff, JoAnn might say something like, "I know this is important to you. I'll see what I can do."

Of course, there were lots of times when nothing could be done. Problems sometimes had to be endured rather than solved; requests sometimes had to be denied.

In those cases, JoAnn would say something like, "I know this is tough for you, but there's nothing we can do right now. Meanwhile, it's important to the whole unit that you hang in there and do the best you can."

Even this registered a Zapp! because JoAnn's people knew that at least their situations had been considered. And they knew their supervisor was with them, not against them.

Flo noticed that responding with empathy seemed to be just as contagious as enhancing self-esteem. It seemed that the more JoAnn responded empathetically to her staff, the more they responded that way to their patients.

When Mrs. Sanders complained that she just *had*

to have regular coffee—"no more of this muddy decaf"—her aide said gently, "I know it's disappointing to have to give up something you really enjoy, but caffeine upsets your stomach. How about some juice or herbal tea instead?"

And when another patient was sitting in the hallway, obviously impatient as he waited to return to his room after some lengthy tests, a nurse spoke to him from where she was working at the nurses' station: "It looks as if you're anxious to return to your room. I can't leave the nurses' station right now, but let me call someone else to help you."

When a patient complained that she was supposed to have some tests done that day, but nobody had come to get her, one of JoAnn's nurses checked the schedule and found out the patient's tests were scheduled for the next day, not today. The nurse said kindly, "I know it can be frustrating to wait all day for tests and then find out they aren't scheduled until tomorrow. I called the lab to see if they could fit you in today, but they couldn't. We did arrange to get you scheduled for first thing tomorrow, though."

Flo noticed that even the patients' families were benefitting from all this Zapping behavior. When Mrs. Sanders was ready to be discharged, Flo saw an aide talking with Mrs. Sanders's daughter: "You sound so excited about having your mother return home. She's really lucky to have such a caring family."

Flo was pleased to report all these happenings to JoAnn, who made a new entry in her notebook.

JoAnn Mode's Notebook

2nd principle of Zapp!:

**Listen and Respond
with Empathy**

15

Some say it came from a long time ago when hospital administrators had tried unsuccessfully to keep it on a leash.

Another explanation was that it had simply existed in the hospital basement for many years—hibernating until awakened by the fanfare accompanying an administrative proclamation of a new hospital policy.

And some say it had grown up at Normal Medical Center—small at first, but growing, slinking about by night, gorging on memos, reports, directives, and other combustibles.

Wherever it came from, it was a big mother dragon. It stalked the Normal Medical Center halls in the 12th Dimension, looking for places to lay eggs. And the field was fertile.

Flo saw it one day while she was experimenting with her newest invention, the Zappometer (pronounced "zapp-aw'-met-er"), which measured Sapp¡-Zapp! ratios and lightning levels.

Over time, the Medical–Surgical unit had become

a much brighter and happier place. In the past week, Flo had observed a 1 to 3 ratio in Sappi-Zapp! frequency, as well as an improvement of 12 bolts in the unit's average Zapp! charge.

Flo watched JoAnn Mode walking through the unit. JoAnn still had her cowboy hat and spurs, but she seldom reached for her six-gun anymore. As she said and did enZapping things—maintaining each person's self-esteem, listening to each person, and responding with empathy—little forks of lightning flashed between her and the others.

Things had improved, but the lightning still did not reach very far or last very long. When JoAnn wasn't around, people got dull quickly. Their glow faded, like red-hot steel cooling down and turning gray. They were still dodging those sticky piles of paper on the floor, and no one seemed too concerned.

Most disappointing of all, not enough Zapp! was getting to the patients. In the Radiology department, the Zapp! connected the staff and the patients, and the charge of energy had become self-sustaining. But in Med-Surg, though there had been some improvements, they had a long way to go.

As Flo was considering the situation, she felt a tremor in the floor. And a moment later another tremor. And another. Then from around the corner came the purple, scaly snout of the dragon.

Like all hospital dragons, this one was invisible to the normal world, but its effects were quite real.

One switch of its tail, and a new regulation would hit JoAnn.

A swipe of its talons, and the data in the unit's computers would be randomly trashed.

A turn of its head, and the entire staff would begin arguing with one another.

Whenever this dragon breathed, crises broke out: equipment breaking down, individual patient needs not even being recognized, doctors yelling at nurses in front of patients, meals arriving late, nurses complaining about the nurses on the next shift.

The dragon squeezed its wings through the hallways of Med-Surg, took a deep breath, and—whoosh—a long stream of red and orange arched across the unit, igniting the visitors' lounge, which burst into a tower of flames.

JoAnn, who had been in the middle of responding with empathy to something Phyllis had said, immediately broke off in mid sentence and rushed to the fire, her cowboy hat bending and twisting as she hurried, until it became a white fire fighter's helmet.

Gladys, an L.P.N. who was closest to the conflagration, had already grabbed a 12th Dimension fire hose and was about to turn on the water, but JoAnn rushed over to Gladys and wrestled it away from her.

Sapp¡—and Gladys's Zapp! charge, such as it was, was grounded.

"Stand aside!" yelled JoAnn. "Everybody out of the way!"

While the flames rose higher, JoAnn stood there figuring out how to turn on the hose.

Meanwhile, the dragon wandered back down the hall toward the Med–Surg nurses' station and flicked its long, forked tongue. The disk in Mrs. Estello's word processor went up in smoke.

As usual, Mrs. Estello had no idea what to do. Her job was to be a unit clerk, and that was all. So, rather hurriedly, she took the smoking disk down the hall to give it to JoAnn who, of course, was too busy wielding the fire hose to pay any attention to Mrs. Estello.

Sappi

Mrs. Estello left, still carrying the smoking disk, and headed for the nurses' lounge for an aspirin. She talked to herself along the way.

The dragon roared again. More red and orange streaked through the air, and another fire erupted on the far side of the unit in the supply cabinet. Then the dragon whipped its tail around to spread the flames.

Now three or four little fires were beginning to burn, and JoAnn was too busy fighting the first fire to notice them. Actually, she was too busy enjoying the challenge. It was fun being a fire fighter. In fact, she was not about to hand her hose or helmet over to anybody else. Why should she? Wasn't this her job?

She just about had the first fire doused when she saw the smoke from the other fires. All of a sudden, fire fighting wasn't so much fun. She tried rushing back and forth among them, spraying one, then the next. But as soon as she turned her back, the fires burned up and up and out of control.

Flo watched, waiting for someone to help JoAnn, but no one did. They were all thinking that JoAnn would know what to do. After all, it was her job. JoAnn might have given them little Zapps now and then, but who were they to face dragons and raging fires? Against those problems, they were still just a bunch of Sapped employees, whirling around the unit like human tops, always on the move but going in many different directions at once.

All but oblivious to JoAnn's heroics, they kept doing what they normally did, or just stood around basking in the heat, while JoAnn ran from fire to fire. And Mrs. Estello, back from the nurses' lounge, tagged along with her charred data disk, waiting for JoAnn to tell her what to do next.

The dragon grinned.

Flo put in a call on the Flo-phone, but JoAnn, of course, was too busy to take it. Later, when Flo came back to the normal world, they finally got together in the old research lab. JoAnn entered the lab as sweaty and tired as a fire fighter could be—and more than a little impatient and frustrated.

"Flo, this Zapp! stuff isn't working," she said. "The patients are complaining, the certification report is late, and Mary Ellen is screaming about the number of empty beds on our unit. We're also behind in turning in our monthly summary because Mrs. Estello doesn't have enough Zapp! to figure out what's wrong with her computer disk.

"The real *monster* of a problem is in the supply cabinet," continued JoAnn, exasperated. "Somebody has been borrowing our supplies and not returning them. We're completely out of IV solution, IV tubing, tape, and dressings. And some of the medications are missing, too. I'll have to take care of this right away."

Placing her hand on her forehead, JoAnn sighed, "I'm too busy solving all the problems around Med-Surg to Zapp! anyone."

After some talking, Flo persuaded JoAnn to take a look at the problems as seen from the 12th Dimension. Reluctantly, JoAnn agreed. After all, what did she have to lose?

By the time they arrived in the 12th Dimension, the dragon had had its fun in Med-Surg. It had deposited a few eggs to hatch sometime later, incubated by the heat of smoldering fires, and had wandered on to other units.

Most of the Med-Surg nurses and aides, while showing concern about the dragon's fires, did very little, if anything. Why? Because they were accustomed to their supervisor, JoAnn, solving all the problems. They just didn't feel much responsibility for putting out fires because JoAnn had never given them that responsibility.

It was easy for JoAnn and Flo to follow the dragon's trail. At the end of one hall, a young nurse was wielding a fire hose and trying to organize a bucket brigade. But the other nurses had very little interest in the buckets or in whether the fires were put out. They were too busy filling out reports describing the effects of the fires.

When the nurse was called away to hose down yet another fire, she neglected to tell the other nurses to put the water *on the fire*. And since Sapped people can't think for themselves or make decisions on their own, the nurses splashed the water every which way. They were tripping over the buckets, spilling water, and bumping into one another. All of which was hysterical to the dragon.

Then, from down the hallway, came the siren. It was the administrative fire truck, gleefully driven by Mary Ellen Krabofski herself, trollish as ever, her fire engine-red fingernails curled around the steering wheel.

Riding the truck with her was the C.O.O. and the entire senior management fire brigade. "Fire Expert" was printed in bright, gold letters on each of their slickers.

Mary Ellen brought the truck to a screeching halt and hopped out. The first thing she did was to run over and take the fire hose out of the nurse's hands.

"Gimme that!" she yelled.

Sapp¡

And what did the expert fire fighters do? First, they ran around the truck half a dozen times, chasing everybody away.

Sapp¡ Sapp¡¡

Then *they* grabbed the buckets and started splashing water.

Sapp¡ Sapp¡¡ Sapp¡¡¡

Down the hall from where the fire truck had come, there now came a knight in shining armor on a white horse. He rode up to Mary Ellen.

"Hi! I'm Sir Lancelot, a dragon specialist," he said. "I fight and kill dragons."

"About time you got here," she said.

"Wow, looks like you've got a big one," said the knight.

"We *know* that," said Mary Ellen, gesturing with the fire hose in hand. "Now go slay it, or I'll rust your armor."

Without even pausing to ask anyone where the dragon might be, the knight dropped his visor, lowered the point of his lance, and charged into the smoke. Unfortunately, his visibility was limited by the tiny slits in the visor, and he galloped right past the dragon, spearing a hospital volunteer instead.

Just then, the dragon slipped out the fire escape. It headed down the 12th Dimension path toward the Radiology department, figuring to liven things up for the Radiology staff.

Flo and JoAnn followed at a discreet distance.

Of course, Radiology was not exempt from visitations by monsters and hospital problems. JoAnn and Flo arrived just after the dragon had entered a room where Claire was holding a meeting with some technologists. The dragon huffed and puffed and breathed fire right into the middle of things.

But Claire did not try to solve the problem of the dragon on her own. She did not put on armor and fight the dragon. She did not put on a fire helmet and fight the fire.

At the first whiff of smoke, she turned to the technologist nearest the fire hose and—lightning bolt forming in her hand—said, "We have a problem, and I'd like your help. . . ."

Zapp!

And *that* person picked up the fire hose and figured out how to fight the fire—while Claire pulled the others together into a group and said, "We have a big problem, and I'd like all of you to help. . . ."

Zapp! Zapp!!

The technologists then started talking among themselves about what to do, while Claire checked on the rest of the department. By the time she returned, the technologists had an action plan worked out.

At a nod from Claire, some of them put on fire helmets. Then Claire got them some fire extinguishers, and they went to work on the new fires the dragon was starting.

The rest of the group put on armor and went to

chase the dragon. Unlike many previous dragons, this one was too big for them to slay or tame on their own, but they did succeed in harassing it into leaving.

All this did not take very long, because dragons, as you know, prefer dark and foggy places to lay their eggs. There was too much energy and light in the Radiology department for it to linger or lay many eggs.

Meanwhile, Claire had gone around to the other Radiology technologists and said, "We're trying to solve a problem, and I'd like your help. . . ."

Zapp! Zapp!! Zapp!!!

The technologists filled in here and there for their coworkers so that the regular work got done during the dragon crisis. No patient was neglected.

After it was gone, it was clear that the dragon had not Sapped the Radiology department. With an abundance of Zapp!, it had been a lot like fighting fire with fire. In fact, the Zapp! now glowed even brighter than before, because the staff was charged up by having met the challenge.

Watching it all, JoAnn realized that Zapp! *did* work. She simply did not have enough of it in her unit, and she was not using it fully yet.

Just as JoAnn and Flo were about to leave, the knight charged into the department. Claire Burton had to hurry over and grab the reins before he carelessly speared one of *her* volunteers.

"Whoa!" she called. "May I help you with something?"

"Don't bother me. I'm on the trail of a big mother dragon," said the knight.

"It was here, but we chased it away," Claire said.

"*What*?!" exclaimed the knight. "You dealt with it on your own? Impossible!"

"But we did," she said calmly.

Feeling threatened, the knight said, "Well, you can't do that. You're not allowed!"

Sappi

The knight rode away. But his Sappi was soon overpowered by the Zapp! in the Radiology department. No single Sappi of a mere threatened knight could take away the energy the staff had achieved.

JoAnn and Flo went back to Med–Surg, where JoAnn called the entire unit staff together.

She began by saying, "I'd like your help in solving a problem."

Zapp!

JoAnn Mode's Notebook

3rd principle of Zapp!:

Ask for Help
and Encourage Involvement

(Seek ideas, suggestions, and
information)

16

In the next few days, JoAnn spent most of her time getting Med–Surg back to normal. Well, almost normal. During this time, her thoughts remained on Zapping, Sapping, and the dragon. "What had gone wrong?" she wondered.

So she called yet another staff meeting for the upcoming afternoon. JoAnn started out by asking, "So why are we having so many fires . . . I mean *problems* . . . around here?"

At first, everyone was too Sapped to talk. After a minute of silence, JoAnn nearly threw her hands up and dismissed the meeting.

But, instead, on a hunch, she used the first principle of Zapp! with the group. She told them that she knew they were all well-trained, dedicated professionals; that every day they saw what was going on; and that they probably had some good ideas about what the problems were.

Susan was the first to venture a guess—with which Corinne promptly disagreed, putting forth a theory of her own. Then Richard had an idea and, before long, lots of people were talking.

JoAnn then Zapped some more by listening to what each person had to say. On a flip chart, she made a list of all their ideas about what might be happening.

The group talked about each idea and then tried to decide on priorities. It was hard because there were a lot of problems on the unit. But finally, after some discussion, they chose the problem that should be attacked first: Doing paperwork took too much time, which meant they didn't have enough time for patient care. In fact, the nurses all agreed that many days, half their time was spent with paper, not patients. They decided that they needed to find ways to spend less time dealing with paperwork and more time caring for patients.

"OK, thanks for your input," said JoAnn. "You can go back to work now."

Everybody nodded and walked away. But as they turned their backs, what happened in the 12th Dimension?

Sapp¡

Well, JoAnn Mode came up with a solution (and a brilliant one, she thought) to the problem of paperwork taking too much time. She got clipboards for the Med-Surg nurses so that it would be easier to fill out all the forms.

Well, JoAnn's improvement did help the paper problem, but only a little, and only when the nurses remembered to use their clipboards. But the change did not really make life easier or more pleasant for anyone. In fact, nobody was very interested in whether they had clipboards or not. Soon, new fires spread in the hallways and patient rooms.

JoAnn talked to Flo, because by now JoAnn had come to trust Flo and her opinions.

"Flo, why isn't my brilliant solution working?" she asked.

Flo had a fairly good idea of what was wrong. Indeed, JoAnn had Zapped everyone by asking them to help identify the problem. Then JoAnn unintentionally Sapped them when she took the problem away from them and solved it herself.

"But they can't come up with solutions," argued JoAnn. "It'll be a waste of time. They don't have my experience, my administrative know-how, my grasp of the big picture."

"Oh?" challenged Flo.

"Anyway, coming up with solutions is *my* job, isn't it?"

"JoAnn, the plain fact is that you still have fires out there," said Flo. "Your idea might have been brilliant, but nobody else had a stake in making it work. They didn't own it. You did. It wasn't *their* solution."

Grumbling to herself, JoAnn finally admitted that Flo might be right. She told Flo to go have a look from the 12th Dimension while she talked with her staff again. At this meeting, she asked for help not just in finding the problem, but in coming up with a solution.

It was Shelby, the newest Med-Surg nurse, who

came up with the best idea. Less constrained by this-is-the-way-we-have-always-done-it thinking, she had a fresh perspective and suggested a way to consolidate two of the unit's reports. She also suggested checking with the director of nursing to find out if all the information the unit provided was really necessary. Was it possible they were spending time gathering data that wasn't really useful?

Everyone, even a very surprised JoAnn Mode, knew immediately that Shelby's ideas were great. The other nurses talked in an excited way about their implications. They all agreed her suggestions could help a lot. There were Zapps all around.

"OK, thanks a lot for that great idea. I appreciate your help," JoAnn said. And then, with a wave goodbye, she added, *"I'll take it from here."*

As soon as she said that, Flo, who was watching from the 12th Dimension, saw the lightning, which was glowing brightly among the people in the group, move from them to JoAnn. Once again JoAnn had taken their lightning—stolen it almost—and Sapp¡¡

JoAnn got busy revising the forms in order to implement Shelby's idea. Then she set up a meeting with her boss, Mary Ellen Krabofski, to check into the usefulness of all the various reports generated in Med-Surg.

But when JoAnn talked to the nurses about the changes each of them would need to make, she could see that they were no longer enthusiastic. They just weren't very interested in whether the forms were shorter or not. Or they said they didn't understand the changes. Or they privately came up with reasons why JoAnn's solution wouldn't work. Even though JoAnn had Zapped them in getting the idea, she had Sapped them by uninvolving them in implementing it.

Just then, in the 12th Dimension, the dragon was heard stomping down the hospital's corridors once more. It breathed fire all over the place. After slinking from one department to another, eventually it ended up in Med-Surg. As usual, everyone was too busy—rushing from place to place and bouncing off walls and one another like popcorn at the height of its popping cycle—to help JoAnn fight the fires. So JoAnn put out the fires herself. Again.

At the end of the day, the dragon wandered on, having enjoyed itself immensely.

Flo challenged JoAnn and said, "You know, JoAnn, something isn't right."

"You're telling me!" said JoAnn.

"Don't you remember the very first time we saw Claire Burton? Remember who fought the dragon?"

"It was one of the technologists," said JoAnn.

"That's right," said Flo.

"And do you remember what happened when another dragon showed up?"

"She got together a team to fight the dragon," said JoAnn.

"And do you remember who *did not* fight the dragon?"

"Well, sure," said JoAnn. "It was Claire Burton who did not fight the dragon."

As soon as she said that, she understood. Claire had offered help, but had not taken away from the individual or the department the challenge of fighting the dragon and its fires. She had left the responsibility with them.

At the next staff meeting, JoAnn went over the problem of excessive paperwork, and again the nurses talked about possible solutions. But after they had talked, JoAnn said, "Let's talk about what *you* need to make this work."

This time the Zapp! stayed with the people in the group. They owned the problem, the idea for solving it, *and* the challenge of making the idea succeed.

For a few of the nurses, this was too much too fast. After years of Sapp¡, suddenly having a bolt of lightning thrown at them was very frightening. Their immediate reaction was to try to get rid of it—to brush it off or throw the lightning back to JoAnn and the other nurses.

JoAnn had to react quickly to make sure these fearful nurses did not Sapp¡ themselves. She listened to their concerns and then said some things to maintain their self-esteem and build their confidence. She also instinctively lowered the voltage for these people, giving them smaller bolts of Zapp!, which would not blow their fuses.

Most of the nurses, though, were happy to accept the Zapp! They carried it away with them back to their work, and it flashed and flickered among them as they cared for their patients.

By the time the dragon made its next rounds, everybody knew what to do as soon as its ugly head came around the corner. Rather than waiting for JoAnn to do something, they picked up the new fire hoses, armor, and swords they had asked JoAnn to purchase for them—and went after the dragon themselves.

Things were not perfect, mind you. Corinne kept tripping over her hose. Richard busily dealt with a tiny fire, while behind him a huge one raged out of control. The dragon chasers were very clumsy with their weapons. And through the crisis, poor old Mrs. Estello just kept typing away, wondering what all the excitement was about.

But this day it was the nurses in Med-Surg who had the good time, not the dragon. The fires were put out very quickly. And the dragon soon left.

"We did it!" they all called to one another.

Watching what happened from the 12th Dimension, Flo saw Med-Surg light up like dawn. And that was how JoAnn Mode learned to generate the electric soul of Zapp! on her unit.

JoAnn Mode's Notebook

The soul of Zapp!:

**Offer Help Without
Taking Responsibility for Action**

JoAnn Mode's Notebook

The first three principles of Zapp! . . .

1. Maintain or Enhance Self-esteem.
2. Listen and Respond with Empathy.
3. Ask for Help and Encourage Involvement.

. . . lead to the soul of Zapp!:

**Offer Help Without
Taking Responsibility for Action**

17

As time went on, JoAnn Mode saw a lot more initiative and interest on the part of her nurses and aides. The trouble was, her revved-up staff was charging off in all different directions. There wasn't much of a focus.

The past crises had been exciting for the unit. It had felt, well, kind of like fighting a pitched battle against an invisible dragon—and winning. Lots of the nurses and aides secretly hoped that other problems would occur. After all, weren't health care professionals trained to deal with *crises*? Didn't their training work best in *emergencies*?

Yes, JoAnn decided, they all needed some direction.

And so she wrote in her notebook.

JoAnn Mode's Notebook

- Zapp! does not guide action. It excites action.
- To get the job done, I have to channel the action in the right direction.
  But how?

JoAnn tried holding more staff meetings so that everyone could talk about improvements, but the meetings became another problem, not a solution. The meetings took a lot of extra time, and it seemed that every time JoAnn called a meeting, Mary Ellen Krabofski would just happen to stop by and wonder why the nurses weren't *caring for patients*.

JoAnn tried to explain to her that the meetings were important, but Mary Ellen didn't buy it.

"That's not what we're paying them to do," she complained.

JoAnn was stumped. How could she get the unit—and the individual nurses and aides—to do the right things without having a meeting every couple of days?

For a while, JoAnn let her staff follow whatever initiatives they wanted to take. She thought it would increase their Zapp!

So when Donna came to her and said that she and some other nurses wanted to put up a new bulletin board, JoAnn said "OK" and helped them get the supplies they needed.

The bulletin board turned out well, and Donna and the other nurses received a lot of compliments.

So they decided to put up a few more bulletin boards to advertise hospital events and other items of interest.

JoAnn began to wonder if the unit really needed any more bulletin boards. But she did not want to Sapp¡ the group's initiative, so she said nothing.

Within a couple of weeks, JoAnn noticed that there were bulletin boards on almost every available wall in the unit. They looked great. But she'd noticed something else: Patients were complaining about having to wait too long for nurses to answer their call buttons. The surgeons were complaining that the nurses were never around. The nurses were late in exchanging their reports. And the aides were complaining that they had to take on some of the nurses' work because the nurses were always involved in their special project.

"That's strange," thought JoAnn.

So she decided to talk with Donna.

"Hey, Donna, what's going on here?"

"No time to talk now," answered Donna. "We're

all too busy keeping everything up to date on the new bulletin boards."

"But putting up bulletin board notices is keeping you from caring for your patients," said JoAnn.

"It is?" asked Donna.

"Yes, in fact, I'd say projects like this are pretty low on the list of things you should be doing," said JoAnn.

Donna shook her head, obviously frustrated, and said, "Well, then, why didn't you *tell* us what was important so we wouldn't waste all this time?"

"Good question," JoAnn thought.

To make matters even worse, Flo came in at the end of the day and reported that the unit's Zapp! level was down by 10 bolts, and dropping quickly. It seemed that without a dragon to focus their efforts on, nurses and aides were changing things that didn't need to be changed, solving problems that didn't exist, throwing their energy in a thousand different directions, and Sapping themselves. Worst of all, they were Sapping the patients.

JoAnn thought for a while. "There are so many things we need to accomplish. I don't know what's most important. It seems we're supposed to keep everybody happy—senior management, the doctors, the patients, and their families. Everything is important to someone!" she concluded.

Realizing that the unit needed direction, JoAnn decided to ask for help. She went to Mary Ellen Krabofski to ask if she could offer advice and explain what she expected from JoAnn and her unit.

But all Mary Ellen said was, "If you don't know what your job is, I'm not going to tell you."

JoAnn retreated to her office. If the director of nursing can't give me direction, she thought, then my staff and I need to figure out what's important. We need to come up with goals for our unit.

At the next staff meeting she asked, "What are the key results we want to achieve, and how can we measure our success?" There was a lot of discussion, but they all agreed on one thing: Everything they did should be directed toward patient outcome, patient care, and patient satisfaction.

JoAnn wrote down the top four *key result areas* they agreed on:

- Providing quality care to the patients.
- Improving the unit's efficiency.
- Completing the necessary reports on time.
- Improving the staff's working relationship with the doctors.

The next issue they took up was *measurement*. How would they measure their progress?

Soon it became obvious that some forms of measurement would be easier than others. For example, it would be easy to know if reports were turned in on time.

But they realized that other types of measurement would be more difficult.

How could the unit measure the quality of its patient care? How could the nurses know whether the doctors were happy with their work? What did "efficiency" really mean?

JoAnn and her nurses discovered that it was easier to figure out *what* they should be doing than it was to determine *how* they could measure their progress.

But JoAnn and her staff refused to give up. In meeting after meeting, they wrestled with the challenge, considering each key result area and brainstorming possible methods of measurement.

Finally, they figured out that their first, most important key result area was too broad. So they rewrote it to say:

> Providing timely, quality care to all our patients
> in a manner that maintains the patients' dignity
> and involves them as much as possible in the
> recovery process.

And how would they know if they were successful? What was "timely" care? What was "quality" care? What would be their goals? Well, figuring that out took some time. Some goals couldn't be set until they collected important baseline data. But for most goals, they could make an educated guess with the intention of clarifying the goals as they got used to the measurements.

After each meeting, JoAnn went to her notebook.

JoAnn Mode's Notebook

To channel action, mutually establish the following:

Key Result Areas—the direction we want to go.

Measurements—ways to know we're moving in the right direction.

Goals—ways to tell us if we're there yet.

Just to be on the safe side (because she knew she might need some approvals from her later on), JoAnn ran all the unit's key result areas, measurement methods, and goals past Mary Ellen Krabofski, who was actually quite impressed.

Mary Ellen immediately did some digging in her files and, from way in the back of her bottom drawer, produced a list of things the hospital's administrators considered important to Normal Medical Center. This list had been created in a meeting several years ago, but nobody had done anything with the list—except to file it away.

As she looked over Mary Ellen's list, JoAnn was pleased to see that her nurses' ideas about what was important matched the hospital's list in most areas. Most satisfying was finding out that the hospital's primary focus matched the unit's top priority: quality care and satisfied patients. And where the lists differed, JoAnn now had some additional ideas to take back to her staff.

At the next department meeting, JoAnn shared the hospital's list of priorities with her staff, and they developed new key result areas where appropriate. For example, two of the hospital's main goals were to reduce costs and increase productivity. After the group figured out ways to measure their progress in these areas, they set goals for the current year.

Then JoAnn suggested another idea she'd been considering: How about using the *unit's* key result areas to develop key result areas, measurements, and goals *for each nurse and aide*?

"How would that work?" asked Sandy.

"Each of you would have individual goals that would relate to the unit's overall goals," answered JoAnn. "That way, you'll see how important you are to the overall success of Med-Surg."

"Great idea!" said several nurses. And they began working on individual plans for themselves.

What really got the nurses excited was the idea of *self*-measurement. All the nurses and aides would be able to measure their own progress in different areas instead of having someone else measuring them. They decided that weekly measurements would be the best for most of them, although some preferred monthly progress checks.

Most everyone liked the idea, but they often got stuck trying to come up with self-measurements.

Larry, one of the Med-Surg nurses who held weekly "wellness" education classes for patients, realized that he needed to generate more patient participation in his classes. Occasionally, he had tried to talk less, but he soon reverted to lecturing for most of every class. Now he was determined to increase the patient participation rate, because he knew it was related to the unit's goals of increasing the patients' involvement in the recovery and aftercare process.

But how could Larry measure his progress? He thought and thought, and finally came up with the idea of audiotaping one class per month. He could listen to the tapes and determine what percentage of time he talked, and what percentage the patients talked.

At the beginning, Larry talked 90 percent of the time, and the patients 10 percent. But each month he improved, and eventually he increased patient participation to 50 percent, which was his goal.

JoAnn knew that all her nurses and aides felt proud of what they were accomplishing because they had personal goals . . . to help meet the unit's goals.

For the first time, the staff knew what was important and why it was important. And they knew how
they were doing relative to measurable goals.

That was an enormous Zapp!

JoAnn wrote in her notebook.

JoAnn Mode's Notebook

Continued tracking of progress
toward goals creates Zapp!

Feedback from your supervisor and
others is helpful; self-measurement
is best.

18

Time passed, and indeed things in Med–Surg began to improve. One day, JoAnn was walking down the hall when Richard stopped her.

"How did the patient survey turn out?" asked Richard.

"Oh, OK," said JoAnn.

The next day a couple of other Med–Surg nurses asked, "JoAnn, how's the department doing?"

"Pretty well," said JoAnn.

After that, they quit asking. A few days later, JoAnn noticed that there seemed to be a slacking off of improvement efforts. Flo had been taking her own measurements of the Zapp! levels, and she, too, had found that they were indeed falling off.

"I told them they were doing pretty well. What's going on?" JoAnn asked Flo.

"But what does *pretty well* mean?" Flo chided. "JoAnn, if you were a basketball player, how good could you be if you could never see whether the ball went into the basket? Or what if you had to play every day, but no one would tell you the score? People who are involved in their work want to know exactly how the whole team is doing—and not tomorrow, today."

"I see what you mean," said JoAnn.

By the next afternoon, there were graphs on the walls of the nurses' lounge, showing the progress toward each of the department's goals. Next to the unit's goals, JoAnn had left room for nurses and aides to note their progress toward individual goals, which supported the overall goals.

JoAnn encouraged her staff to post their own progress charts and to keep them up to date. Some were reluctant at first, but eventually most of the staff posted their charts in the lounge. After a few months of developing confidence that the charts were designed to help them, not get "evidence" against them, some of the staff decided to share their goals with the doctors and patients, so they posted them outside the nurses' station. Soon, everyone was doing it.

Very quickly, JoAnn saw that sharing the measurement methods and goals had an amazing effect. Nurses and aides started helping each other—sharing "tricks of the trade" learned through experience. They took pride in one another's accomplishments, and they were supportive when there was a temporary downturn in the data.

Because they could see what their coworkers were trying to accomplish, there was more cooperation around the unit.

At first, JoAnn and her staff tracked what they'd

been told to measure by the Quality Assurance department—things like blood usage, medication administration variances, and patient falls. But then some of the staff came up with ideas about other areas of measurement that would be even more useful in providing timely, quality care—things like how involved patients and families were in the planning of their care, and how well individual needs were being met.

JoAnn and her staff soon found that measurements were very helpful—but only if they were measuring the right things and only if the data was timely, accurate, and complete.

JoAnn made another note in her notebook.

JoAnn Mode's Notebook

Measurement focuses attention on what is important and tells the team how it is doing.

The three vital areas of measurement are:

- Timeliness
- Accuracy
- Completeness

Patients noticed that the staff was setting and tracking goals, and knowing the nurses' and aides' goals made the patients feel encouraged by the unit's high standards. Some of the patients even decided to try to help the staff reach their goals.

For example, Larry found that his patients asked more questions in class after they learned about Larry's goal for increased patient involvement. They also began suggesting topics for his weekly classes: They wanted to know more about nutrition and special diets, family support groups, stress-reduction techniques, and mental health.

What JoAnn hadn't expected was that some of the patients wanted to set their own goals and chart their own progress. Patients who were going to physical therapy sessions, for example, wanted to chart things like strength and endurance. This really excited the patients, and the Zapp! level continued to increase.

At first, most of the surgeons scoffed at the idea of posting charts all over the unit. JoAnn even heard a few of them grumbling among themselves that the Med-Surg nurses were only asking for trouble by displaying all this data for the world to see.

One of the surgeons, Dr. Lee, though, was a bit more open-minded. "Let's see if it does any good," he suggested to his colleagues. "The nurses and patients seem to be benefitting from it. Who knows, maybe in time we'll all benefit from it."

And indeed, Dr. Lee was right. Several months after the charts went up in the halls, he overheard one of the other surgeons admit, "I'd been thinking about sending my patients to another hospital, but now I'm referring people here more than ever before. My patients and their families have been raving about the nurses and aides."

It took time, but eventually some of the other doctors got into the act, too. Why? Because they recognized that all this Zapp! stuff was really working! They saw that their goals needed to be part of the department's goals. And once they took on their new challenge with enthusiasm, there was a lot more collaboration between doctors and nurses and more support of one another. Doctor-nurse teams sprouted up, and doctors and nurses began to feel more involved in one another's successes, all of which helped to improve patient care.

Despite JoAnn's fears—and the doctors'—about showing "bad news" on the charts, they discovered that sometimes even this could be a Zapp! How could that be? Because the staff tried a little harder if they saw they were falling behind.

And if someone continued to fall behind, nobody had to be the bad guy in saying something about performance being off. The measurements told the story.

From the unit's experiences with measurements, JoAnn learned an important lesson: You can change people's focus by changing what they measure. This was so important that JoAnn decided to make an entry in her notebook.

JoAnn Mode's Notebook

Managing by Measurement:

- Continuous tracking of progress toward goals keeps the Zapp! level high.
- Changing measurements and goals Zapps people in new directions.
- One of the most effective things a nursing supervisor can do is to change the measurements to reflect what is most important.

Most of the time, the measurements on the graphs went up, up, up. And within a year, Med-Surg was reaching or exceeding most of its goals.

19

When JoAnn and her staff first began surveying Med-Surg patients about their satisfaction with the unit, they had expected to find the patients most impressed with the state-of-the-art technology and procedures. But to their surprise, they found that what made patients feel most satisfied—or dissatisfied—was *how they were treated*.

This led the Med-Surg unit to realize that patients have two kinds of needs: practical and personal. The *practical* needs were those related to their medical conditions—things like receiving their meds on time, having the necessary tests completed, getting adequate rest, and receiving good information. The *personal* needs were those related to simple, common courtesy; being treated with dignity and respect, and having some control over what was happening to them.

Because JoAnn's staff was well trained technically, they found that meeting the patients' *practical* needs came easily. But meeting and exceeding the patients' *personal* needs took more practice.

"Maybe the staff needs some training on using the

key principles," thought JoAnn. "I see them being used, but not all the time and not by everyone." So at the next staff meeting, she presented the key principles as a way of meeting patients' personal needs. After they discussed examples of how each principle could be used, everyone agreed to try them out with their patients.

As JoAnn and her staff practiced using the key principles, they found that the first two principles—*maintain or enhance self-esteem* and *listen and respond with empathy*—worked beautifully. But when they tried to use the third key principle with their patients—*ask for help and encourage involvement*—it was more difficult.

For example, one day Ruth was talking with a patient about his frustration at having to stay in the hospital longer than planned. After Ruth maintained his self-esteem, and listened and responded with empathy, she asked the man for his help in solving the problem.

"How can *I* do anything?" the man answered. "You're all in charge here, not me!"

Ruth realized the patient was right: His attending physician had ordered the longer hospital stay because he felt it was important for his patient's recovery. So asking the patient to help solve the problem didn't seem to be the answer.

So Ruth tried asking for help in areas the patient could control. "I know it's disappointing to have to stay in the hospital longer than you'd planned," she began. "But if we work together, I'm sure we can make your time here pleasant and beneficial to your recovery. Why don't you tell me what ideas you have for accomplishing that."

Well, that did it! The patient brightened up and was even eager to discuss his ideas for making the next few days worthwhile.

But he didn't have many ideas because he didn't know what was available in the hospital. So Ruth made a few suggestions, and then they talked about all the ideas they both had come up with.

Ruth had learned something valuable, so she shared it with JoAnn and the rest of the unit at their next meeting: They needed to adjust the third key principle when dealing with patients. Ruth suggested, "Ask for ideas and/or offer suggestions."

The group liked Ruth's idea and decided to post their "Key Principles for Patients" in the nurses' lounge as a reminder that these principles were *key* to providing service beyond patient expectations:

Key Principles
for Patients

1. Maintain or Enhance Self-esteem.
2. Listen and Respond with Empathy.
3. Ask for Ideas and/or Offer Suggestions.

As JoAnn Mode and the Med-Surg nurses, aides, and volunteers used their revised key principles with patients, they saw wonderful results. For example, Sandy, a nurse who previously had shown a tendency to be rude to patients, learned that she provided much better service when she took the key principles with her on her rounds. As she became better at using the key principles, she also found that she was enjoying being a nurse again. It wasn't just a *job* any more; it was a profession in which she could make a real difference in people's lives.

JoAnn, who knew how rude Sandy *used* to be, simply beamed when she saw her one day talking with a patient. Sandy was saying, "It's time for your treatment, but I see you have visitors. If you're comfortable enough to wait, I'll come back after your visitors leave. Or, if you'd rather ask your visitors to step out in the hall, it shouldn't take long. Which would you prefer?"

Zapp!

That same day, JoAnn overheard Sam, another nurse, talking with a patient about a request that Sam couldn't grant. The patient wanted to take a shower, even though his doctor's instructions clearly said "no showers" for another day. Sam explained why the shower was not advisable at this time, but the patient was clearly disappointed.

Normally, Sam might have said something like, "You can't take a shower until tomorrow. That's the doctor's orders." But remembering the key principles, Sam said instead, "I can tell you're disappointed, and I understand your frustration. It's hard not being able to shower. How about a sponge bath today, and I'll make sure you get to shower first thing tomorrow morning?"

Zapp!

JoAnn also saw her staff using the key principles in dealing with the patients' families. For example, when a patient's wife wanted to talk with her husband's doctor in the evening, instead of in the morning when Dr. Marcus made his rounds, the attending nurse, Carol, explained that an in-person, evening conversation with the doctor wasn't possible. But the wife kept insisting.

Finally, Carol decided to ask for the woman's help in solving the problem. Carol said, "Well, it seems we have a problem here. It would be more convenient for you to talk with the doctor in the evening, when you come to visit your husband, but Dr. Marcus is here only in the mornings. Do you have any ideas about how we might resolve this problem?"

To Carol's surprise—*pleasant* surprise, that is—the woman calmed down and suggested that if she could meet with the doctor early in the morning, she wouldn't have to be late for work. Carol knew that there was a staff meeting at 8 A.M. the next day and that Dr. Marcus would be there. So she suggested a 7:45 A.M. meeting and offered to make the necessary arrangements with Dr. Marcus.

"I'd really appreciate it," said the woman.

"Well," smiled Carol, "I'm glad to help."

Zapp!

One of the aides, Nan, was especially good about

meeting or exceeding the needs of her patients' family members. When asked for directions to a nearby hotel by an out-of-town visitor, Nan could have said, "It's right up the road. You can get directions at our information desk down in the lobby." But instead, Nan said, "The easiest way is to go out of the parking lot and turn right. Follow the signs to Route 79, and then take Exit 12. The hotel is on your right."

Nan's willingness to help with directions had certainly met the man's needs. But then Nan added, "If you'd like, I could draw you a map or walk down to the lobby with you and point you in the right direction." When Nan offered this extra help, she exceeded the visitor's needs by going above and beyond the call of service.

Zapp!

Things were truly going well, but JoAnn noticed that some people still needed more guidance in meeting patient needs. They could use the key principles, but not always resolve the problem. Some sort of road map was needed.

After some thought, JoAnn decided to add the topic to the agenda of the next staff meeting.

At the meeting, they discussed the need to define some steps for meeting patient needs, and they appointed a committee to suggest appropriate steps.

The committee decided that the most direct way to get an answer was to ask some of the more experienced nurses how they handled situations. And so they did just that.

The senior nurses were only too happy to help. In fact, they were pleased to be recognized for their experience.

The committee got a lot of good ideas and came up with four steps that seemed to handle most situations. They summarized these at the next staff meeting.

The first step, they decided, was to *acknowledge* the patient's situation or request—to show the patient that you recognize help is needed.

Second, they had to *clarify* the situation to make sure the patient needs are understood.

Third, they would do everything possible to *meet or exceed* the patient's need.

Fourth, they would *confirm the patient's satisfaction* by asking, "Does that meet your need? Is there anything else I can do?"

After a rousing discussion, all agreed on the four steps. JoAnn and her staff left the meeting, knowing that they had accomplished something very important: They had developed a plan of action for meeting or exceeding their patients' needs.

Before leaving work that day, JoAnn made sure she entered the plan in her notebook.

JoAnn Mode's Notebook

Steps to follow in meeting or
exceeding a patient's needs:

1. Acknowledge the person.
2. Clarify the situation.
3. Meet or exceed the need.
4. Confirm satisfaction.

One Monday morning, JoAnn was walking around
the unit when Corinne told her about an unusual situation that had occurred over the weekend.

Within only a short time, JoAnn learned of an
extraordinary service effort by an aide, Tammy. One of
the Med–Surg patients had been in the hospital for
more than two months. Although the man's condition
was terminal, he was able to be discharged.

During his stay, the patient had lost a lot of weight.
When the patient found out he was going home, he
wrote to his son, who lived out of state, and asked him

to send him some new clothes in smaller sizes. The clothes arrived two days before the man was to be discharged. Everything fit fine, except that the pants were much too long.

When Tammy was talking with the patient about his medication, she asked if there was anything he was concerned about or needed before leaving the hospital. He hesitated a moment and said, "Well, no. Everything's fine. You've been so helpful." The aide asked a few more questions and found out about the pants.

Tammy offered to take the pants home and hem them herself. Then she brought the pants back the next day, hemmed and pressed. On the morning the patient was leaving the hospital, he waited until Tammy came on her rounds so that he could show her how well the new pants fit. He thanked her again, and then said good-bye before leaving the hospital.

JoAnn knew her nurses and aides were providing excellent service to the Med–Surg patients now, and that made her happy.

There were times, of course, when a patient or a family member was so upset that they didn't want to talk about alternative solutions. They just wanted to express their anger or frustration. They needed to let off steam and, until they did, the steps for meeting patient needs didn't work. The individuals needed someone to hear them out and show an understanding of why they were so upset.

At one of their staff meetings, the Med–Surg group came up with a clever way to remember that in these circumstances, the effective thing to do was "take the heat" before dealing with the issue. JoAnn thought their ideas were so good that she wrote them in her notebook.

JoAnn Mode's Notebook

Remember, when all else fails, take the **HEAT**:

Hear them out.

Empathize.

Apologize.

Take responsibility for action.

One of the nurses at the staff meeting was concerned about how to apologize to patients. "In some cases, because of possible legal ramifications, we should be careful not to admit fault," she pointed out.

"You're right," said JoAnn. "We should *apologize for the situation without accepting blame.*"

"For example," JoAnn explained, "you might say, 'I'm sorry for the inconvenience' or 'I'm sorry you're upset.' "

"Or 'I apologize for the breakdown in communication,' " suggested Larry.

"Good example," said JoAnn. "And remember not to go overboard in apologizing. If you go into too much detail about problems or mistakes, it could make the hospital appear incompetent."

Then the group discussed *taking responsibility for action.*

"If you can resolve the problem on the spot, then do so," explained JoAnn. "If you can't resolve the problem immediately, then take some action to show the patient that something is being done."

"For example," JoAnn continued, "you could call a supervisor or the appropriate department, or take notes and offer to follow up on the problem later."

"In other words," suggested Flo, "we should do whatever we can."

"Right," said JoAnn.

No one in Med-Surg liked to "take the heat." But

they knew that sometimes that was all they could do. There was no turning back the clock to prevent something from happening that had already occurred. And so they took the heat and helped their patients feel as good as they could.

After a few months, JoAnn saw that providing outstanding patient care was also helping to meet the goal of increasing the number of filled beds on her unit. Why? Because the satisfied patients leaving Med-Surg were telling their doctors—and their families and friends—about the wonderful people who worked in Med-Surg.

For example, JoAnn heard a patient say that she'd talked with one of her neighbors, Mr. Schwartz, a former patient in Med-Surg. Not only had Mr. Schwartz's surgery gone well, but he'd been especially happy with the care he'd received in Med-Surg. One nurse in particular had listened to his fears, spent time with him explaining all the procedures, and even held his hand on the way to the operating room.

Remembering her conversations with Mr. Schwartz, the new patient said, "I didn't think twice when my doctor asked me which hospital I'd prefer. My neighbor had told me so many good things about his experiences here that I'd never go anywhere else."

JoAnn walked away, wondering how many *other* people had heard Mr. Schwartz's story. She was proud of her staff. They definitely were feeling more lightning, and the patients were beginning to feel more lightning, too.

JoAnn realized that she had learned something important: *Good service meant good business.*

She wrote in her notebook.

JoAnn Mode's Notebook

Excellent patient service . . .

- Not only satisfies our current patients . . .
- But also attracts new ones.

20

Great things were happening in Med-Surg.

And how did JoAnn Mode feel? Did she feel like a hero? Did she feel terrific?

No, she began to feel more and more nervous and scared.

Flo noticed the change.

"JoAnn, what's wrong?" she asked. "You look worried. You're not Zapping people the way you could be. What's holding you back?"

JoAnn muttered some feeble excuses, but Flo kept pressing her until she admitted what was really bothering her.

"To Zapp! people in a big way, I have to encourage them to get more involved and take on more responsibility, right?" asked JoAnn.

"Right."

"But if I let other people take responsibility, how do I know they'll live up to it?"

"I guess you have to trust them," offered Flo.

"Trust them? That's easy for you to say. Most of

the time, things go pretty well, but remember when I tried letting everybody make their own decisions? It was a disaster!" said JoAnn.

"That's true," Flo agreed. "But that was a long time ago. Aren't things better now?"

"Of course," answered JoAnn. "But I feel as if I should monitor what's going on. What if things don't get done on time? What if somebody does something I don't know about and everything gets messed up? Who is Mary Ellen Krabofski going to yell at?"

"You," admitted Flo.

"Right. Me. I'll get yelled at. I'll get the blame. And if the mistake is bad enough, there's no telling what could happen to me," said JoAnn. "Sure, I'd like people to be Zapped—but not if it's going to get me in trouble."

"Look, you Zapped me when you asked for help figuring out how Claire ran the Radiology department. You gave me responsibility. Did I let you down?" Flo argued.

"No, but I knew what you were doing," said JoAnn.

"Well?"

Had you been in the 12th Dimension, you would have seen a new sun rise inside JoAnn's head. Of course! Offering help to people on the unit partly meant staying in touch with them, knowing what they were doing and what they planned to do, and keeping them on track.

In short, there still had to be some sort of monitoring and coordination. But how could she keep track of people's activities without Sapping everyone?

Within five minutes, JoAnn had everything she needed to figure it out.

The phone rang, and it was a new nurse, Debra, who was having trouble with a member of the Respiratory Therapy staff. She was comfortable caring for patients—in fact, she was quite good at it—but she was very uncomfortable *handling problems with other departments*.

JoAnn thought back to her early days as a nurse. She had been unsure about handling problems involving other departments, too, but now it was a routine part of her job.

"How about if I role-play the situation with you before you meet with the person? That will give you some practice, and maybe I'll be able to give you a few pointers," offered JoAnn.

"That would be great," said Debra, relieved. "In fact, that's just what I need—a good coach!"

All of a sudden, the bells went off in JoAnn's head. Of course! Debra needed more of JoAnn's help because she was new to nursing. She needed more coaching and more frequent checks than an experienced nurse.

And that's when it hit her: Monitoring, in the sense of knowing what's going on, didn't have to be a Sapp! It could be a Zapp! It all depended on the situation and the person.

JoAnn figured out that monitoring was largely a

matter of how often she should check on how her nurses and aides were doing and how she did the checking. Repeated coaching and checking up on experienced staff would be a Sapp¡ and a waste of time. But coaching and checking up on a new employee, or an employee experiencing difficulties, would be a Zapp! because it showed concern—and this certainly would be an excellent way for a unit supervisor to spend her time.

JoAnn also learned that there were many different ways of knowing what was going on. Of course, direct observation was important, as were periodic written reports on progress and one-to-one meetings with her staff. But far less threatening was "management by exception." People were told that they needed to inform her only when measurements passed a prearranged trigger point—like the time the response rate for treatments went down, not up, and JoAnn felt the need for more information.

Most important, JoAnn discovered an extremely effective way of monitoring was just to walk around and talk with people. This way, she found out what was going on, and she had the opportunity to throw a few Zapps into the conversation.

It took some practice, but JoAnn finally got the hang of it. She learned that instead of looking over everyone's shoulder, she could help employees *as they needed it*.

This was an important thing to remember, so JoAnn wrote it in her notebook.

JoAnn Mode's Notebook

A nursing supervisor needs to know what's going on in the unit—with nurses, aides, support staff, and volunteers. Observations, periodic written reports, and meetings are effective methods of monitoring—but so is just walking around.

The best way of knowing what's going on is to coach people.

- A supervisor who *over*monitors Sapps.
- A supervisor who *abandons* monitoring Sapps.
- A supervisor who uses *situational* monitoring Zapps.

People respond negatively to monitoring only when it is inappropriate for the situation.

With practice, JoAnn also learned that she could share responsibility with her staff without their thinking she was abandoning them. Through Zapp!, the Med–Surg staff took on new responsibilities, and that was good.

JoAnn could see that her role was changing, but it was as important as ever.

She went to her notebook.

JoAnn Mode's Notebook

My role as a nursing supervisor is changing. But I still have the responsibility to:

- Know what is going on.
- Establish direction for the department.
- Ensure that everyone on the staff is on course.
- Make the decisions that the staff can't.
- Offer a guiding hand and open doors to clear the way.
- Help to assess performance.
- Be a smart supervisor . . . and a good coach.

21

Unfortunately, Mrs. Estello was still making mistake after mistake with hardly a break.

One day JoAnn went over to her and pointed out this fact. She tried to be as patient as she could as she said, "You see, the problem is that for our unit to reach its new goals, we're going to need your help in reducing the number of mistakes in the work coming from your area."

Mrs. Estello nodded vaguely and looked as if she might be thinking about an unpleasant side effect of something she'd eaten for lunch.

"You've been doing this job for a long time," JoAnn continued. "I'm sure that with all your experience, you can think of ways you might improve your accuracy."

"I can?" she asked.

"Sure you can! Just give it a try. We'll talk about it on Wednesday, and if there are things you need, let me know," said JoAnn.

She went away thinking that surely Mrs. Estello would respond to what she had said.

The next day, Mrs. Estello was still making all kinds of blunders. In fact, JoAnn learned that 10 boxes of syringes had arrived on the unit, when the nurses had asked for 10 boxes of bandages—all because Mrs. Estello had hit the wrong code key on her computer and never looked back.

Just about everything coming from Mrs. Estello had to be done over again, and by Wednesday her performance had gotten worse instead of better. The nurses and doctors were complaining to JoAnn more than ever about Mrs. Estello's work.

So JoAnn talked with Mrs. Estello again.

"Why do you think you're making so many mistakes?" she asked.

"I don't know," answered Mrs. Estello.

"How could you improve?"

"I don't know."

"Didn't you come up with any ideas like we talked about?" JoAnn asked.

"Not yet. I haven't had time," said Mrs. Estello.

After work that day, JoAnn was telling her husband, Joe Mode, what had happened.

"She's hopeless! She'll never get it! Never in a billion years!" JoAnn complained to Joe.

"Maybe you're asking too much too soon from Mrs. Estello," Joe suggested.

"But I have tried to coach her. It works for other

people, but not for her. She's holding back the whole unit!" JoAnn cried. "I should fire her!"

"It sounds as if you're really upset," said Joe. "Why don't we take your mind off work for a while? Let's go out in the backyard and see what the kids are up to."

JoAnn figured that was a good idea.

When they got outside, they found their young son, Jack, and their daughter, Jill, trying to play baseball. They watched as little Jack Mode flailed away at the ball his older sister was pitching.

After his fourth useless swing, little Jack turned and said, "I can't do it!"

"Sure you can," said Joe Mode.

"But I don't know how!"

So Joe stepped down from the porch and worked with little Jack.

First, he talked with little Jack to make sure he understood the object of the game. Then they talked about important details: how Jack had to keep his eye on the ball, when to swing, and how to choke up on the bat to get more control.

Next, Joe said, "Now watch me." And he took the bat and showed little Jack how it was done.

Then he gave the bat to Jack and said, "Here, you try it now."

Which Jack did. The ball came across the rock they were using for home plate, and little Jack swung the bat—and missed.

But, being a good father, Joe Mode did not yell at him. He just said, "Good swing! Now try it again.

You'll get the hang of it. Keep your eye on the ball."

JoAnn watched as he had Jack practice—over and over again.

Finally—CRACK!—little Jack connected and sent the ball rocketing over the back hedge.

"See, you're a natural!" called Joe, as his son ran for the brick that represented first base.

Of course, little Jack was *not* a natural baseball player. He had succeeded because his father had taken the time to coach him and because he had practiced. And, as his parents watched proudly while little Jack ran the bases, JoAnn suddenly realized where she had gone wrong with Mrs. Estello.

She had expected too much too soon, and she hadn't been a good coach.

Just as she would never tell her kids, "If you don't hit the ball the first time, you're out of the family," it wasn't right for JoAnn to demand too much of Mrs. Estello without helping her to live up to her expectations.

The next day, JoAnn approached Mrs. Estello and said, "Mrs. Estello, I'm going to work with you on this. Maybe if we put our heads together, we can figure this out. Now first, let's talk about what we're trying to accomplish. . . ."

By and by—working not only with Mrs. Estello, but with others as well—JoAnn found that there were seven basic steps to being a good coach on the job.

First, she had to establish the overall purpose of the

task and explain why it was important—how it related to achieving the unit's goals or the individual's goals.

Then she had to explain the process to be used in accomplishing the task.

Next, she had to demonstrate how the process was done or have someone else provide a demonstration.

Then JoAnn had to observe while the person practiced the process.

She had to provide immediate and specific feedback, and then coach again or reinforce success.

JoAnn had to express confidence in the person's ability to continue to accomplish the task successfully.

And finally, they had to agree on follow-up actions—in other words, how they would measure progress.

For example, through coaching, JoAnn tried to keep Mrs. Estello from making mistakes in the first place. In other words, JoAnn coached her for success. When a new project was assigned, she coached Mrs. Estello so she would *start out* doing it correctly.

JoAnn found that Mrs. Estello learned much faster when she coached her before the start of a project instead of after she had made some mistakes. That way, Mrs. Estello never had a chance to learn bad habits or get frustrated by the mistakes she was making. Coaching made a new project exciting and challenging.

One day, for instance, Mrs. Estello came up with an idea for increasing productivity on the unit: She wanted to change her working hours so that she would arrive on the unit an hour earlier than the professional staff. That way, she'd get a "jump start" on the work for the day. "While her idea might have merit," JoAnn thought, "I wonder how it would affect the unit at the *end* of the shift. . . ."

JoAnn decided the thing to do was to *coach for success*. So she offered support and encouragement to Mrs. Estello in investigating the option of starting her shift an hour earlier every day. For example, she suggested ways Mrs. Estello might find out what the rest of the unit thought about the idea and helped her determine who else in the medical center she should check with. With clear direction, and coaching from her supervisor, Mrs. Estello was on her way.

JoAnn Mode's Notebook

To get maximum Zapp!, people need to be coached on how to do their jobs.

Coaching steps:

1. Explain the purpose and importance of what you are trying to teach.
2. Explain the process (the steps) to be used.
3. Show how it's done (model the behavior).
4. Observe while the person practices the process.
5. Provide immediate and specific feedback (coach again or reinforce success).
6. Express confidence in the person's ability to be successful at the task.
7. Agree on follow-up actions.

JoAnn found that the more she coached for success up front, the less she had to coach for improvement later on. As she worked with Mrs. Estello and others in Med-Surg, JoAnn learned how to make coaching a regular part of her job.

JoAnn saw that coaching gave Mrs. Estello the confidence to try new tasks, like using a new software program recommended by Data Processing. Soon, JoAnn learned that it wasn't a lack of ability holding Mrs. Estello back from trying new things nearly as much as it was a lack of confidence in herself. Her successes built confidence, which led to more successes, which led to more confidence.

Zapp!

JoAnn Mode's Notebook

People learn faster from successes than from failures.

It still took time for Mrs. Estello to improve, but she did. In the meantime, JoAnn asked the other staff members dealing with her to help come up with some ways to lighten Mrs. Estello's load, which they did.

As JoAnn worked with Mrs. Estello, she discovered that very little of the information Mrs. Estello was processing was meaningful to her. What required immediate attention and what didn't? What was related to what? Mrs. Estello did not know.

So JoAnn chose some of the most commonly requested reports and arranged for Mrs. Estello to talk with the people who received these reports. Mrs. Estello found out how the information was used and why it was important. During this process, she even found that one report she'd been spending an entire day every month to complete wasn't used any more—so she stopped producing it altogether.

JoAnn also spent time talking with Mrs. Estello about the expectations for a unit clerk. Little by little, she expanded Mrs. Estello's universe.

Zapp!

JoAnn Mode's Notebook

Learning more about your job boosts
your Zapp!

When Mrs. Estello did something wrong, JoAnn
would take her aside and explain what was wrong and
show her how to correct the problem. Every time Mrs.
Estello did something right, JoAnn made sure she knew
about it. She told Mrs. Estello why it was right and
talked with her about what she had to do to *keep*
getting it right.

She would say things to Mrs. Estello like, "Your
work has been a lot more accurate lately, which helps
the entire unit. I'm really impressed."

Zapp!

Still, it was not a steady climb for Mrs. Estello.
From time to time, she would get angry at JoAnn for
asking her to do things that she didn't want to do. Or
she would become defensive about her performance.
Or she would get the idea that JoAnn was manipulating
her, and her trust in her supervisor would weaken.

Then Mrs. Estello would slip back into her old ways and attitudes.

For example, Mrs. Estello had a tendency to take longer lunch breaks than scheduled. When JoAnn realized that the problem was getting worse, not better, she knew that she had to say something.

"Mrs. Estello," JoAnn began. "You are a key player in our group. We all rely on your reports, and so do a lot of other departments. It's important for you to be at your desk during regular hours so we can get the information we need. I noticed you were gone over the lunch break longer than normal last week. How can I help you keep on schedule?"

Then JoAnn talked with Mrs. Estello, listening to her comments and discussing suggestions for solving the problem. Mrs. Estello agreed to reschedule some of her noon commitments for after work so that she could be back from lunch on time, and she thanked JoAnn for helping her see why this was important.

"Wow!" thought JoAnn. "It worked!"

JoAnn thought back to other times when she'd had to deal with personnel issues and poor work habits on the unit. It seemed that the longer JoAnn put off talking with someone about a problem, the harder it was to approach the person—and the harder it was to correct the problem.

With Mrs. Estello, though, JoAnn had dealt with the issue in a timely way. And she had remembered to focus on the problem, not on the person, offering to help in any way she could. *Together,* JoAnn and Mrs.

Estello had come up with workable solutions. And because they were both on the same side, both had "won" when the problem was solved.

JoAnn wrote in her notebook.

JoAnn Mode's Notebook

Putting off dealing with personnel issues only makes them harder to resolve.

Confronting personnel issues as soon as they surface allows a nursing supervisor to focus on coaching for improved performance—and it's a lot easier to get a "win" for both parties.

JoAnn learned that the most valuable tools for getting Mrs. Estello back on track were the key principles. JoAnn remembered to maintain or enhance Mrs. Estello's self-esteem, listen and respond with empathy, ask for help in solving problems, and offer help without taking responsibility away from her.

Sure enough, Mrs. Estello continued to improve.

And it was working with other people on the unit, too.

Zapp!

JoAnn Mode's Notebook

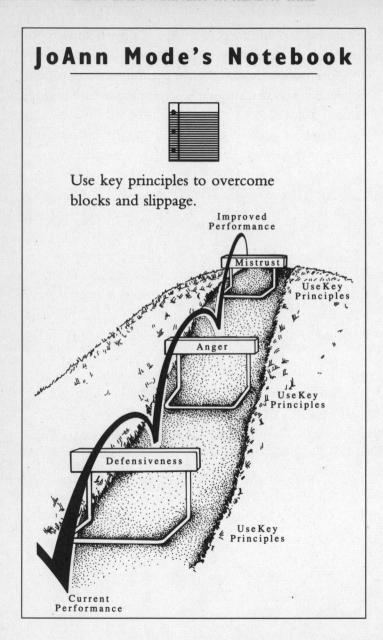

Use key principles to overcome blocks and slippage.

JoAnn also discovered that being a good unit supervisor meant following up on performance discussions—especially if the person's performance had not improved. JoAnn came to the conclusion that her goal in such follow-up meetings would be to spell out the consequences should the person fail to correct the problem—and then come up with a workable plan to get the person back on track.

This type of discussion was difficult, admitted JoAnn to herself. But using the key principles made it easier.

In time, JoAnn decided that all her hard work was worth the effort because, sure enough, she saw real improvement in the unit—especially with Mrs. Estello. Mrs. Estello *herself* asked for some additional computer training.

Zapp!!

Then, based on her training, Mrs. Estello learned how to set up her keyboard so that she could create a whole paragraph just by hitting one key. And she asked JoAnn for a software program to check her spelling. She wanted to be *accurate*!

Zapp!!

Then she figured out how she could type an entire form by selecting from half a dozen keys that filled in the blanks automatically.

Zapp!!!

And before long, Mrs. Estello was not hopeless. She was good at what she did.

She was a glowing member of Med-Surg's team.

22

Month after month, JoAnn could see that not only was the unit changing, but her role as a nursing supervisor was changing as well. She was no longer the supervisor she used to be.

For years, JoAnn had believed that she knew just about everything there was to know about being a nursing supervisor. In her own mind, she had seen herself as a lieutenant in the Army of Health Care.

To be a good lieutenant, she was supposed to:

Follow orders from above.
Make all the decisions for her "troops."
Keep everyone under control.
Be tough and unapproachable.
Bark orders at people.
Yell at people who did something wrong.

Yet this approach no longer worked (if indeed it ever really had) in the Med–Surg unit. Something had long been missing.

What she had learned was that her position required her to be less like a tough boss and more like a good parent. When JoAnn was growing up, her parents had helped her grow from being a helpless child to a responsible member of the family. Slowly they involved little JoAnn and her brothers and sisters in running the household. They gave them more and more responsibility and decision-making power as they grew up.

Of course, JoAnn knew that her nurses and aides were adults and not children, but she knew that the same ideas—growth, involvement, increasing freedom with increasing responsibility—applied to adults, too.

Her job was no longer a matter of ordering the staff around. Her job was to supply what they needed to provide excellent patient care and to grow professionally and personally.

And what was it that Zapped people needed?

First, they needed *direction*. It was JoAnn's job to make sure her staff worked on the right things. She did this by establishing key result areas, measurements, and goals.

Second, they needed various types of *knowledge and skills*. For example, they needed ongoing professional training, personal skills such as problem solving, and an understanding of how the entire hospital system operates.

Third, they needed their supervisor to help them get the necessary *resources*—equipment, materials, facilities, time, and money.

Fourth, they needed JoAnn's *support*—encouragement, authorization, coaching, feedback, recognition, and reinforcement.

Instead of trying to be a solitary "hero," JoAnn Mode—like Claire—was giving her staff whatever was required to let each of *them* be the "hero." She gave whatever was needed, and her unit gave back their personal best.

JoAnn Mode's Notebook

For Zapp! to work, people need:

• Direction (key result areas, goals, and measurements).

• Knowledge and skills (advanced technical training, interpersonal and problem-solving skills, and an understanding of how the system operates).

• Resources (equipment, materials, facilities, and time).

• Support (encouragement, authorization, coaching, feedback, recognition, and reinforcement).

All this was fine with JoAnn. She liked her position better this way, and her staff seemed to like their assignments better. Yet, something was bothering her.

One evening she told her husband, Joe, "You

know, I don't seem like a *supervisor* anymore. The title doesn't fit. I'm not *looking over* people now."

"So what do you do in your job now?" Joe asked.

"Well, I point out to the staff which direction we have to go in, and I guide them so they get there on their own, but with no one straying too far off the path. That way, we all get there together," explained JoAnn.

"To me," said Joe, "that sounds like the job of a leader. You're not directing as much as you're leading a group."

"To lead the group," JoAnn thought, *"rather than direct the group."*

She sat back and tried to imagine her name linked to a new title:

JoAnn Mode, Unit Leader

"Hmm," she mused. "I kind of like that."

And the Zapp! grew.

JoAnn was walking around Med–Surg one afternoon when she passed Richard, who told her about a patient complaint he had heard that morning. But JoAnn was not to worry about it, for it was not a problem anymore—because Richard had already handled it on his own.

As JoAnn was walking by Room 324, she noticed that Gladys was visiting with Mrs. Watson, a patient who had been clinically depressed since breaking her hip several weeks before. Mrs. Watson's extended stay in the hospital, combined with severe pain and a slower-than-expected recovery, had almost resulted in her giving up on getting better.

But ever since Gladys had decided to stop in to see Mrs. Watson for a few extra minutes every day, JoAnn had noticed an improvement in Mrs. Watson's mood. Knowing that Gladys cared enough to stop in and see her every day was making a difference. And as Mrs. Watson's depression began to lift, JoAnn could see that her physical recovery was speeding up, too.

Just then Phyllis hurried up to JoAnn. She had just completed a revised schedule for the unit and wanted to show her boss. JoAnn could see that Phyllis was very proud. And the schedule looked like a real improvement.

As JoAnn passed a group of ambulatory patients, they all smiled and spoke to her. They were happy, and JoAnn felt good, because all was *not* normal in Med-Surg. It was much better.

JoAnn was especially pleased to learn that a group of nurses had done something to help an elderly man who had been in the hospital for some minor emergency surgery. He was to stay in the hospital recovering for two days. The patient, who had an easygoing and humorous personality, was well liked by all the nurses and aides in Med–Surg.

During her rounds on the patient's last day, one of

the nurses said, "Well, I bet you're looking forward to leaving." But the man didn't look happy at all. Instead, he looked upset and said, "I don't know why you people are in such a hurry to get rid of me."

The nurse talked with him for a while, asked some questions, and found out that he didn't have a home to go to. Just before his surgery, there had been a fire in his fixed-income apartment building, and the repairs wouldn't be finished for another couple of days. He couldn't afford a hotel, and he had no family in the area.

The nurse explained the situation to some of the other nurses, and they decided to take up a collection. They gathered enough money among themselves and other hospital employees to get the man a hotel room for a few days.

They also talked with Social Services to find out what type of help might be available for him through local agencies.

The next day, as the man was leaving, JoAnn saw that he was smiling again. He waved good-bye, thanking everyone for their kindness.

JoAnn looked around, amazed. The Med-Surg staff members were acting like owners of their work, and they were proud of what they did. Things were not perfect on the unit, and probably never would be. But they were a lot better, and sometimes they were fantastic. The employees and volunteers had a sense of who they were, liked it, and knew they were important to their patients.

JoAnn was pleased with what she had heard and seen. As she sat down at her desk, she thought about her new role as a unit leader. And indeed, she felt like a *leader*!

23

At the end of her shift, JoAnn was relaxing in her office when she realized that it had been a long time since she had seen what things looked like from the 12th Dimension. She suspected things would look different from what she remembered, so she decided to find Flo and hitch a ride on the Flo-Vision.

When JoAnn got to the old research lab, all was quiet. Flo was not there, but a note on the door read:

JoAnn decided to join Flo in the 12th Dimension. By now, Flo had installed menu-driven software for the Flo-Vision, which made it easy for JoAnn to figure out which commands to enter.

She double-clicked the computer mouse. There was a high-pitched whine, a blinding flash, and then JoAnn Mode vanished.

When she opened her eyes, JoAnn saw the Med-Surg unit surrounded in a light she had never seen before. The fog and mist had lifted. As she walked around, it was as if the sun had come out, except that the sun was inside the doctors, nurses, aides, volunteers, and patients.

In the shadowy corners, there were still some dragon eggs, and nothing could be done at the moment to dislodge them. But JoAnn remembered when it had been different shades of gray.

As JoAnn looked around, she saw no more whirling human tops, no more mummies.

Everybody in Med-Surg was growing into exactly what they were—*human beings*.

JoAnn was extremely happy with what she saw.

But Flo was nowhere to be seen, and JoAnn wanted to talk to her.

JoAnn decided to see if Flo might be in the Radiology department. She left the bright lights of Med-Surg and found her way through the still-foggy hallways in the rest of Normal Medical Center.

She passed the mother dragon, who was wreaking havoc in Pediatrics but who, oddly enough, seemed a bit smaller than when JoAnn had seen her last.

She passed more dragon eggs, huge piles of sticky papers, and lots of other strange sights. Finally, she arrived in the Radiology department.

But where was Flo? Not in Radiology. So JoAnn went back into the fog and checked a few more places, but Flo was not in any of her usual haunts.

As she kept looking, JoAnn roamed farther and farther through the fog. Pretty soon, JoAnn gave up, but when she tried to go back, she realized she was lost.

For a while, she wandered around haphazardly. She happened down a winding staircase, into a courtyard, and through a wide archway flanked by a massive set of gates, where a bored security guard stood leaning on his 12th Dimension spear.

On the far side of the archway, JoAnn realized that she was *outside*. In fact, she was standing on the planks of what she came to realize was a drawbridge.

And there, standing in front of her on the far side of the moat, were Flo Knight and Claire Burton.

"Hi, JoAnn!" called Flo.

"Pretty wild, isn't it?" said Claire, smiling.

"What are you two doing here?" asked JoAnn.

"Flo has been showing me around," said Claire. "In fact, we were watching you for a while. I was picking up a few pointers."

"You were?" asked JoAnn, feeling proud.

"I think it's time we compared notes, don't you?" asked Claire.

And they did just that.

24

As experts on the subject now agree, there are two ways to enter the 12th Dimension. The first is by sitting in the swivel chair wired to Flo Knight's Flo-Vision. The second is to bump into someone by accident who is already in the 12th Dimension.

Which was what Claire Burton had done.

Flo (invisible, of course) had been in the 12th Dimension, with Zappometer in hand, as she wandered over to the Radiology department to have a look at a new kind of lightning she had noticed.

Claire had been hurrying toward her desk to take a phone call when Zapp!—she slammed right into Flo, was drawn into her field, and vanished from the normal world of three dimensions.

When her eyes adjusted, Claire found herself in the land of lightning bolts and strange yet brilliant visions. And here was this Med-Surg nurse saying, "Oh, hi!

Gee, I guess you'd like to know where you are and what's going on, wouldn't you?"

"Yes, please," said Claire, hands covering her pounding heart.

So Flo decided to give Claire the grand tour. That was what they were doing when JoAnn Mode showed up.

Well, once she heard what had been going on, Claire could have been a little upset that JoAnn had not approached her and been more open about things. But Claire was more interested in this new way of looking at how the different units in the hospital *really* operated, and she was even *more* fascinated by the power of Zapp!

"All these years I've been trying to create this, without ever knowing if it really existed," said Claire. "And now I can actually see it!"

"But what are you doing out *here*?" JoAnn asked them.

"It occurred to me as I was showing Claire around," answered Flo, "that I had never looked at the entire medical center from the perspective of the 12th Dimension. So we came out here to take a look."

"Look at that courtyard in the middle of the castle," said JoAnn. "What's that?"

They all turned toward a large field surrounded by parts of the castle. The field was sectioned off in squares that were separated by huge stone walls.

"So each unit has its own maze. That's interesting," said JoAnn.

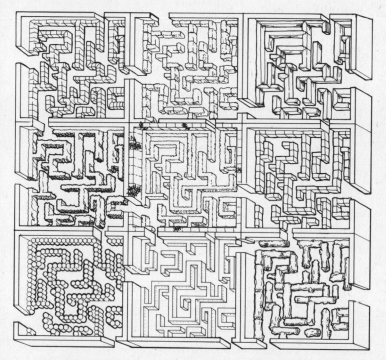

Overlooking the entire Normal Medical Center was a high tower on which flew the Board of Directors' flag. The tower seemed to be growing as they watched.

"But where is the Med–Surg unit?" asked JoAnn, who wanted to know (as Claire had before JoAnn had arrived) where her own unit stood in the scheme of things.

"It's over there. Don't you see it?" asked Flo,

pointing to a tower on the left side of the building.

JoAnn finally saw where Flo was pointing. The glow of lightning bolts could be seen through the windows.

Then JoAnn noticed that unlike the other towers, which had narrow, rectangular windows, this tower—their tower—had little *round* windows.

And *fins*.

It also had a smoother, sleeker shape than the other parts of the castle.

This tower seemed to be much more *fluid*.

As JoAnn scanned the sight before her, there, on the far side of the outer walls, she saw another tower, also with fins and little round windows in the walls. And behind the windows, the lightning of Zapp! flickered and glowed.

It was, of course, the Radiology department.

These two towers were different from the others. Something extraordinary was taking place.

JoAnn could see that they were no longer shapes of set stone, but shapes transforming, evolving into something new.

PART III

Super-charged Zapp!

25

Well, they all found it very interesting to see the medical center this way, but it was time to get back to their units and get ready to leave for the day. So the three of them returned to the worlds of Med–Surg and Radiology. In parting, there were lots of promises to talk often and keep in touch.

But those promises were never kept.

In days to come, they were all much too busy with their own units.

Claire Burton did visit Med–Surg a couple of times, and she asked to use the Flo–Vision so that she could do some exploring on her own.

And then lots of people from the Radiology department took trips to the 12th Dimension. Not just the staff, but radiologists and volunteers as well.

This miffed JoAnn Mode a bit. People coming in and out were a bit disruptive, and they were making demands on Flo's time.

But this was a minor irritation. JoAnn Mode had lots of other things to keep her occupied. Chief among them was the task of trying to keep everyone Zapped.

One afternoon on her way home, JoAnn finally admitted something to herself that she really didn't want to: As time went on, she was finding it harder—not easier—to keep her nurses, aides, volunteers, and patients Zapped.

JoAnn was using everything she knew, but she could not get the kind of quantum improvement in involvement and performance that she had been getting before. Zapp! as she would, JoAnn even found the overall lightning level falling off just a little. And she knew it even without Flo telling her the exact measurements.

"What else can I do?" JoAnn asked herself as she drove home one day. Then she shrugged and said, "Well, maybe we've reached our limits. Maybe this is as good as it gets."

About a week later, Flo entered JoAnn's office, carrying a copy of *The Normalburg News*. "Hey, JoAnn," asked Flo, "have you seen this?"

On the front page was a story that read:

Normal Medical Center's Radiology Department Receives President's Award for Reducing Costs and Providing Outstanding Patient Care

Normal Medical Center's director of nursing, Mary Ellen Krabofski, congratulated Claire Burton, radiology supervisor, and her staff for receiving the President's Award of Excellence. In a ceremony at Normal Medical Center, the unit received a wall plaque and a $150,000 award. Claire Burton said the money will be used to continue research on improving processes within the Radiology department.

"The Radiology teams deserve all the credit," said Burton. "Their hard work, enthusiasm, and creativity are what allowed us to overcome many *hurdles* and enrich the quality of patient care. The cost savings is an extra benefit of our efforts to streamline our processes. I'm quite proud of the Radiology department staff. Because of their commitment, our patients are the real winners!"

"An award?! What's going on over there?" asked JoAnn.

"I don't know," said Flo. "I figured we were doing as well as they were, so I haven't been checking on them lately."

"Well, fire up that machine of yours, and let's go find out what they're doing," said JoAnn.

When they got to the Radiology department in the 12th Dimension, everything looked about the same as usual. Claire was walking around in her wizard hat, and the usual miraculous things were going on. But then Flo started getting a very strong reading on her Zappometer.

"Look at this, JoAnn. The Radiology department is running at 100 bolts an hour!" exclaimed Flo. "The best we've ever done is 75."

"How could that be?" asked JoAnn.

"What can I say?" asked Flo. "The Zappometer does not lie."

"Where's the Zapp! coming from?" asked JoAnn.

Flo moved the Zappometer around to try to determine direction. "It's coming through the windows!" said Flo.

They looked out and saw a strange kind of lightning. It was coming from a group of technologists and volunteers who were huddled together at the end of the maze.

JoAnn and Flo moved closer to the new lightning and, as they did, the Zappometer went off the scale.

But they didn't need an instrument to tell them they were seeing something different from the usual Zapp! they were accustomed to seeing. This was a *wheel* of lightning, flashing among the people as they talked.

JoAnn and Flo noticed other differences, too. The

team members had posted directional arrows along the optimal paths of the maze, making it easier for patients to get through. They also had created maps that they were handing out at the beginning of a patient's entry to Radiology. Both the directional signs and the maps were making it a lot easier for the patients who, Flo and JoAnn noticed, were moving faster and seemed to have fewer frowns on their faces.

Then they noticed that the Radiology team had moved out of the huddle to clip away at the hedges connecting several of the pathways, making the journey through the maze a lot easier and faster.

As JoAnn and Flo watched in amazement, the wheel of Zapp! ran round and round among the team members, going in both directions at once, and back and forth over the diameter of the group, seeming to gain more momentum by the minute.

The kind of Zapp! that Flo and JoAnn had been used to seeing in the 12th Dimension was mostly the simple, linear kind. That is, it sparked from the person in charge to the person reporting to the person in charge—from JoAnn to Flo or from Flo to one of her patients. It did not go round and round, from one person to the next, and back and forth through the group.

But this Zapp! did.

"So what is it?" asked JoAnn.

"Gee, I don't know," said Flo. "It must be because

they're working as a team. I've been reading a lot about teams in my nursing journals."

"But what could be enZapping about teams?" JoAnn wondered. "We've all tried teams before. All of us in Med–Surg are a team. We have patient care teams. And I'm on the hospital supervisors' team."

"What I want to know," said Flo, "is what's making it happen? Claire is way over there. She isn't even here to do the Zapping!"

That was the other very unusual thing about this type of Zapp! It seemed to have no single source, but instead was generated by the group itself.

JoAnn watched the wheel of Zapp! and knew that there was more to Zapp! than she understood. Could Zapping people in teams be the next step?

It wouldn't be difficult to set up some staff teams, JoAnn reasoned. JoAnn went over her list of nurses, aides, and volunteers in Med–Surg and divided them into teams. The next day, she told everybody which teams they were on and assigned team leaders. Then she asked Flo to monitor what happened. JoAnn was expecting great things.

A few days later, Flo announced that the Zapp! count had indeed risen: It was now up to 76 bolts per hour instead of 75.

"Is that all?" asked JoAnn, obviously disappointed. "OK, Flo, I'd like your help in finding out why our teams aren't generating more Zapp!"

After some investigating, Flo determined that the

teams were not really teams at all. The Zapp! still flowed from JoAnn to each team member, not around and among the team members in the group.

"You might be calling them teams," said Flo, "but the staff and volunteers have no more sense of involvement than if they were just a bunch of people working in the same unit. They're teams in name only."

"Then how come the teams in the Radiology department are enZapping and ours are not?" JoAnn wondered out loud.

Immediately, the phone rang.

"Because our teams aren't normal work teams," said Claire Burton when JoAnn Mode answered the call. "Our teams are Zapped!"

26

"Where are you, Claire?" asked JoAnn Mode.

"I'm in the 12th Dimension, talking on the Flo-phone. I was just checking up on my own performance, and I could see that you were trying to involve your people in teams and not getting very far," Claire said. "You know, we really should talk more often."

"You're right. We should," agreed JoAnn, knowing that Claire was right.

"I've set up teams, but I'm hardly getting anything for my trouble," continued JoAnn, obviously discouraged. "What type of teams do you have?"

"Well," answered Claire, "we have project teams that take on specific assignments, like the problem we had communicating to other departments about changes we were making in some of our procedures—so we wouldn't have a lot of people confused or frustrated. The project teams handle specific projects."

"We also have ongoing teams like our quality improvement team made up of radiologists, technologists, and volunteers. They meet every month to brainstorm ideas, review regulations, and suggest ways for us to improve," Claire explained.

"But we have those, too," said an exasperated JoAnn.

"Our teams are different, though," Claire explained. "They're . . . well, for lack of a better term, they're *Zapp! Teams.*"

"What do you mean?" asked JoAnn.

"There are a lot of things that groups of people can do better than individuals working alone," Claire answered, "because everyone brings unique ideas, experiences, and information. But the biggest difference is that you can give a Zapp! Team more authority than you can give an individual."

Claire continued: "For example, you usually can't give an individual employee the authority to recommend new equipment, but you can give a *team* of employees that responsibility. Teams are a great way of increasing the Zapp! level."

"Aha!" said JoAnn, who now understood that Zapp! Teams were another extension of the same path her unit had been following—which was away from Sappi, toward more decision making by those nearest the situation.

After she and Claire hung up, JoAnn went to work.

First, she asked for help from the doctors and her staff in setting up new teams instead of trying to impose *her* setup on them.

Zapp!

The teams created by the Med–Surg unit grew out

of the basic functions and responsibility areas of the unit. They were organized so they had all the people needed on the teams to make decisions for an assigned area. Once the teams were formed, JoAnn, as the overall unit leader, worked with each team to establish its key result areas, ways of measuring success, and specific goals. It was important for the teams to know what they were to accomplish and what their limits of authority were in meeting goals.

Zapp!!

JoAnn worked hard to give the teams the necessary authority to make meaningful decisions. For example, she allowed one team to make decisions about defining accountability in specimen collection and defining protocols for medication administration. At other times, the team's function was to come up with meaningful recommendations to present to JoAnn. Either way, though, JoAnn made sure that everyone understood how each team's key result areas fit in with the overall result areas of the Med-Surg unit and—beyond that—with the overall key result areas of the medical center. In this way, the teams felt involved and knew that their time was being spent meaningfully.

Zapp!!

JoAnn had learned a lot, so she made an entry in her notebook.

JoAnn Mode's Notebook

Some things to remember about a
Zapp! Team:

- A Zapp! Team is different from
  other kinds of teams.
- A Zapp! Team is more productive
  and creative than a group of Zapped
  individuals.
- Teams that help supervisors make
  decisions (participate) create small
  amounts of Zapp!
- Teams that are responsible for
  significant job-related decisions
  create high levels of Zapp!
- Creating teams spreads Zapp!
  throughout a hospital unit.
- To reach super Zapp! levels, a
  hospital unit team must be allowed
  to make some of the decisions
  previously made by unit supervisors.

Notebook ▤ (cont'd)

- Teams provide an opportunity to Zapp! people who are difficult to Zapp! as individuals because of the nature of their jobs.

27

At first, the project teams took on relatively easy challenges. For example, one team came up with a simple solution to the problem of people borrowing equipment and not returning it. They gave everyone small cards with a hole punched in one end and put a hook next to where each piece of equipment was stored. Anyone taking a piece of equipment simply hung their name card on the appropriate hook.

Another team of aides tackled the problem of wasted meals on the unit. It seemed that many times after a patient was discharged, meals for that patient kept arriving on the unit, only to be returned to the hospital kitchen—and then eventually thrown out. The team suggested that a copy of all discharge papers should be sent to the dietician immediately upon the doctor's discharge orders. In this way, Med-Surg could bring the dieticians into the communication loop and avoid wasted food and wasted time sending meals back to the kitchen. Not too long after the unit began copying the kitchen staff on all discharge papers, one of the dieticians called JoAnn to tell her how well the new system was working.

In time, ongoing teams were formed to address three important issues: reducing medication errors on the unit, decreasing the amount of time elapsed between cases in the operating room, and improving medication delivery within the unit.

The team of nurses given the responsibility of reducing medication errors on the unit started off with a bang. They knew that Normal was required by regulation to collect data on medication errors, but no one did much with the data. They reasoned that improvements could come about if people were more aware of the amount and types of errors.

"It seems we need several kinds of information," suggested one of the team members. "What kind of errors occur, how often, and on what shift."

First, they checked with JoAnn to see if it would be acceptable to post medication errors.

"Yes," JoAnn explained. "It's appropriate for us to post our performance in order to help us improve our process. On the other hand, we don't want to alarm our patients or 'advertise' our errors. What ideas do you have?" The team took it from there.

One of the nurses figured out how to put all the data on one chart. The team posted the chart inside the nurses' station and explained to the staff how to interpret the data.

It took a while to get everyone on the unit used to checking the chart, but eventually people got the hang of it. Some of the staff didn't like seeing a graph of the unit's mistakes, but in time, they came to understand that they couldn't make improvements if they didn't know where and when the errors were occurring. The chart also allowed everyone to see the impact of improvements being made.

After six months, the team was happy to report that Med–Surg's medication errors had been reduced by 25 percent.

The second team, assigned to decrease the amount of time elapsed between cases in the operating room, was also busy. Early on, this team of nurses had decided it would be helpful to get a surgeon's input on the kind of information that should be tracked to determine causes of slow down and to monitor improvements. Knowing how supportive Dr. Lee had been in the past, the team approached him about becoming a member of the team.

"I'd be delighted," said Dr. Lee. "Decreasing time between cases in the operating room is very important. I'd suggest you focus on measuring on-time starts for the first case of the day and time between cases."

"That's very helpful," said one of the nurses. "Should we also measure on-time anesthesia administration?"

"Yes," answered Dr. Lee. "That's another good idea."

After the team started to get good, reliable data, they were able to implement some easy solutions that showed immediate improvements. They also began tackling more difficult areas. They seemed to be off to a good start.

And how was the third team progressing?

Not very well, JoAnn discovered.

Tasked with the goal of improving medication delivery within the unit, this team of nurses and aides was stuck. How could they improve delivery of prescriptions to the unit, they wondered, when Pharmacy was so slow?

One day when JoAnn checked in with the team to see how things were going, she found that the team members were caught up in a blaming mode. It was obvious that the nurses and aides were very frustrated.

"We order meds as soon as we get the doctor's orders," began a nurse, "but it takes forever to get a prescription filled. Then the doctors and patients blame us for the delay. It isn't fair."

"That's right," said the other nurse. "It isn't our fault, it's Pharmacy's."

"Sometimes the prescriptions even get lost," continued one of the aides. "It can be a real mess. And just try explaining a lost prescription to a patient or a doctor!"

JoAnn decided it was time to intervene.

"Is it possible," she suggested, "that the problem is

no one's fault? Could it be that our current system just doesn't work?"

"Well . . ." said one of the nurses, "maybe so."

The nurse then elaborated: "The doctors write their prescriptions on the patients' charts. But because so many people need to see the charts, the prescriptions don't reach Pharmacy until hours later—or, sometimes, not at all. I guess when that happens, it isn't fair to blame Pharmacy."

"It seems we've learned something: We should be focusing on how to improve things, not who to blame," said the team leader. "We really got off track."

"But you're back on track now," JoAnn pointed out. "And that's what's important."

"What if we developed a form specifically for the doctors to fill out for prescriptions?" suggested one of the aides. "That way, the doctors' instructions for prescriptions could go straight to Pharmacy."

"Good idea!" said the team leader. "Our team could create the form, and then we could show it to the doctors and Pharmacy to make sure it meets everyone's needs."

"That's a great approach!" said JoAnn, pleased to see that the team really was on track now.

JoAnn went to her notebook.

JoAnn Mode's Notebook

- Blaming other departments doesn't solve problems.
- Examining processes does!

28

In the 12th Dimension, JoAnn observed something strange about her teams. When they started out, only small bolts of lightning would pass among a few team members. As the teams got organized and started accomplishing things, though, more and more bolts were exchanged.

But the lightning did not automatically include everyone. Some people were left out. At other times, instead of lightning, sparks would fly, and the Zapp! level would plummet. Then the teams would have to start over again to build up any amount of voltage.

JoAnn decided to take a closer look, and so she sat in on some team meetings. She observed that some people would dominate meetings, doing most of the talking and pushing the group to accept their ideas. Some members weren't participating at all because they weren't at ease speaking up. Other team members tried to participate, but people wouldn't pay any attention to them. Teams sometimes broke into factions or cliques that diverted the meeting from its intended purpose.

And often the teams jumped to conclusions about a problem before exploring alternatives. As a result of their haste, not everyone had the opportunity to give input. JoAnn could practically see a big black cloud of Sapp¡ forming over the dispirited team members' heads.

Occasionally, people got really angry or upset. One day, a team member started to cry about the way her ideas were being ridiculed by another team member. In another team, a member quit, declaring that attending meetings was a waste of valuable time because the team wasn't accomplishing things fast enough. Situations like this would often set back the progress of the team. In fact, it was almost like starting over.

When the Med-Surg teams ran into trouble, everyone blamed the team leaders—individuals chosen by their fellow team members to coordinate team activities. It was *their* job to make *their* teams effective—wasn't it? Team members assumed little responsibility for team functioning. And when the team leaders didn't know what to do, nothing happened.

At first, JoAnn thought only the team leaders needed training. She reasoned that if they did their jobs effectively, they would keep the meetings on track and help everyone participate. But that didn't work. It turned the teams into one-person shows—the team leaders' shows.

In time, JoAnn learned that *everyone* needed training in both team leader and team member skills. Leadership in a Zapp! Team did not rest only with the team leader. It was shared among team members who all take responsibility for different items on the agenda, according to their assignments.

To assume this new responsibility, team members had to learn new "people" skills—how to interact with one another, how to work things out among themselves when egos and personalities clashed, how to hold effective meetings, and how to solve problems as a group. They also needed to learn to value diversity among their members and to support one another, even when there was disagreement.

JoAnn often had to go to Mary Ellen Krabofski for the training resources her teams needed, and Mary Ellen was not always the most receptive boss in the world. Sometimes she would approve JoAnn's requests with a handshake and a smile, and other times—out of habit—she would give her a cranky and gruff rebuff.

But as JoAnn Mode's parents used to say, "Where there's a will, there's a way." Because JoAnn had the will, she almost always found a way to get what her teams needed.

As always, JoAnn kept her notebook up to date.

JoAnn Mode's Notebook

Training boosts the voltage of Zapp!
Teams:

- All team members should be trained in member *and* leader skills.
- The most important skills needed are:
  —People skills for interacting with one another. (This includes training about the key principles.)
  —Holding effective meetings, resolving conflict, and valuing differences.
  —Solving problems, making decisions, and involving others in decisions to get their input and buy-in.
- Unit leaders must provide ongoing coaching and support if the training is to be effective.

Early on, JoAnn learned that it was important to allow adequate time for training sessions. This was tough, because everyone was always busy. But JoAnn worked with her staff to *make* time for ongoing training, which had become a top priority—and another key result area—for the unit.

As they became more confident and better trained, the Med-Surg employees working on Zapp! Teams began to get involved in making new kinds of decisions. For example, they decided when and where they would meet, what problems the teams would tackle, and what criteria would be used to evaluate their performances.

The Med-Surg teams' responsibilities expanded. But because the responsibilities were shared by the group, every team member had partners to count on.

JoAnn was so pleased by the progress of the problem-solving teams that she decided to create a team to take on some of her administrative responsibilities, such as shift assignment, vacation scheduling, and delegating specific responsibilities. At first, some of the team members were reluctant to assume those responsibilities, but with a lot of encouragement and coaching, they agreed—and they succeeded!

JoAnn continued to learn from the teams and added to her notebook.

JoAnn Mode's Notebook

In addition to making job-related decisions and solving problems, teams can be responsible for making governance decisions like:

• Determining work schedules.
• Deciding who gets trained in what.
• Allocating resources.
• Ordering supplies.

When one of the Med–Surg teams decided to look for more efficient ways to handle starting patients' IVs, they came up with what they thought would be a simple improvement for a simple problem. The problem, as the team saw it, was that patients had to wait too long for a nurse to start their IVs because only some of the nurses on the unit handled this procedure. The value of the idea seemed obvious: If *all* the Med–Surg R.N.s started IVs, then the patients wouldn't have to wait as long for the "right" nurses to be available.

The team reasoned that their improvement would allow patients to have their IVs started sooner and make all the R.N.s feel good about being able to handle this procedure. So they asked JoAnn if they could hold a brief staff meeting to share their recommendation.

At the meeting, the team told everyone that they had figured out a way to improve the current system for starting IVs. From now on, they told the Med-Surg staff, all R.N.s would handle this procedure.

"Sorry," said Corinne, "but I won't start IVs. You can count me out."

"Me, too," said Sam. "No IVs."

The team members looked at one another in surprise. What was the matter with Corinne and Sam? Didn't they see that this recommendation was perfect?

"What's the problem?" they asked Corinne and Sam.

"I'm not comfortable starting IVs," answered Corinne. "I haven't done it in so long, I've lost the touch."

"Me, too," answered Sam. "I was trained a long time ago."

"Oh," said the team members. "We didn't think about that."

"Maybe," suggested JoAnn, "the team could look into what would be involved in getting retraining for our nurses who haven't started IVs in a long time."

"OK," said the team leader. "I guess we didn't spend enough time *assessing the situation*."

So the team went back to the drawing board. They found out that the lack of refresher training was indeed one of the reasons more Med–Surg R.N.s weren't starting patients' IVs.

So they decided to come up with a list of several possible solutions for consideration by senior management and the cost of each. When they got all their facts, they asked JoAnn for her help in setting up a presentation to senior management to get approval for the necessary retraining. Because of their well-researched presentation, they got the approval.

Eventually, all the R.N.s in Med–Surg were starting IVs, and the timeliness problem improved significantly.

The team had learned a number of important things: not to jump to conclusions about problems or solutions, not to determine solutions until they had defined the problem, and how important it was to involve others in order to reach the correct decision and get acceptance of the decision from those involved.

The team decided that what they needed was a step-by-step approach that would keep them on track as they worked their way through a problem.

After much discussion, the group came up with a system for attacking problems and opportunities. They were so excited about their design that they called a special unit meeting.

At the meeting, JoAnn watched proudly as her

team members—more Zapped than ever—handled the presentation without relying on her.

"Why not?" thought JoAnn. "It's their idea. They own it. It's theirs to share."

And share they did—not only their decision-making system, but the recognition for developing it. There were Zapps everywhere, and they weren't coming from JoAnn.

JoAnn watched and listened as nurses Zapped doctors and doctors Zapped nurses. The aides and volunteers also got into the act, enhancing one another's self-esteem as they shared credit for the *team's* idea.

A light bulb went off in JoAnn's head as she realized a new discovery: Her staff could Zapp! one another! Zapping could happen sideways! It didn't have to come from the unit leader! She realized that that's what creates the circle of Zapp! she had seen in the Radiology teams.

With this realization, JoAnn was positively Zapped herself!

Suddenly, JoAnn realized that she'd been so busy watching all the Zapps flying around the room that she'd forgotten to pay attention to the presentation. She focused her eyes on the speaker just in time to hear her conclude.

" . . . and using this approach can help us pinpoint the actions we need to take to reach a correct decision and get it implemented. That's why we call it the *Action Cycle*. Using it will help ensure that our improvement efforts are efficient and successful. The cycle focuses not just on coming up with good ideas, but on planning the implementation of the ideas.''

At that point, the team's Action Cycle was unveiled. And JoAnn, who was now taking her notebook to all her meetings, included the Action Cycle among the ideas she didn't want to forget.

Everyone liked the Action Cycle, and all agreed that training on its use should be included in the team training programs that were being coordinated.

JoAnn Mode's Notebook

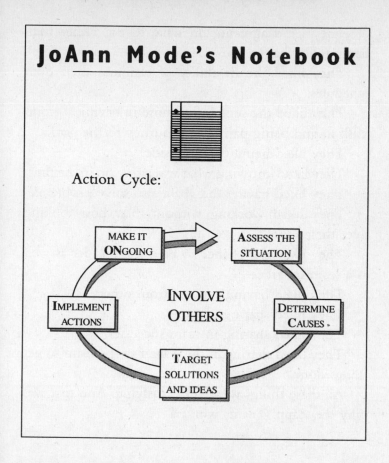

Action Cycle:

MAKE IT
ONGOING

ASSESS THE
SITUATION

INVOLVE
OTHERS

IMPLEMENT
ACTIONS

DETERMINE
CAUSES

TARGET
SOLUTIONS
AND IDEAS

Time passed, and JoAnn continued to monitor the team. She found that most of the Med-Surg staff didn't like *everything* about teams. But they soon realized that the disadvantages of being on a team were more than offset by the advantages of having teams.

For instance . . .

They liked having a voice.

They liked agreeing on what to do, rather than being told what to do.

They liked the flexibility of planning their own schedules.

They liked the sense of purpose in having a group mission and being part of the journey to the goal.

They liked being on the inside.

They liked knowing what was going on in the unit.

They liked having the chance to solve problems.

They liked working without their boss looking over their shoulders.

They liked the chance to be a team leader as well as a team member.

They liked having support from others.

They liked sharing ideas.

They liked sharing in team successes.

They liked sharing in the power of the team to get things done.

All these things were very satisfying. And that was why the Zapp! Teams worked.

JoAnn Mode's Notebook

Why Zapp! Teams work:

1. Communication
2. Involvement
3. Creativity
4. Mutual support
5. Shared ownership
6. Commitment
7. **Empowerment**

PART IV

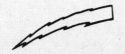

Healing the Processes

29

As you might imagine, things were going pretty well in Med-Surg now that Zapp! Teams were part of the unit. JoAnn and her staff were proud of their accomplishments, and morale just kept getting better and better.

One day, though, as Flo and JoAnn were talking, they realized that for several months now, the Zapp! "temperature" of the unit had remained the same. The Zapp! Teams were still taking on new challenges, the doctors and other hospital employees seemed happy, and patient care indices were at an all-time high.

But JoAnn wasn't satisfied, and neither was Flo.

"There's still something missing," thought JoAnn out loud. "Our people love their jobs. They come to work every morning glad to be here and looking forward to caring for our patients. The doctors and nurses are working together more closely than ever before. And our aides and volunteers really feel like an important part of the team."

"You're right," said Flo. "Things have never been

this good before. The Zappometer ratings have never been so high."

"But they've been steady now for a long time," continued JoAnn. "Surely there's even *more* we could be doing."

"But what?" asked Flo.

"I don't know," admitted JoAnn. "But we'll figure it out. I know we will."

Just then, JoAnn had a thought.

"Let's go back to the 12th Dimension!" she suggested.

"You read my mind!" answered Flo. "I haven't cranked up the old Flo-Vision in quite a while."

So off they went, hoping to discover a cure for whatever was ailing the Med-Surg unit and keeping it from reaching new heights.

As JoAnn and Flo wandered around Med-Surg in the 12th Dimension, they were pleased to see a lot of changes. Nurses, aides, and volunteers were still moving around at a quick pace, but they weren't dodging huge stacks of sticky papers everywhere they went. True, there were still papers scattered around the unit. But the piles were smaller, and they were stacked neatly against the walls.

Flo and JoAnn also noticed that there were no papers blocking the doorways to the patients' rooms. The pathways were clear so that all the health care providers could get to their patients quickly, unimpeded by the papers that used to be *everywhere*. People were still jumping or crawling over hurdles as they moved through the halls, but there were fewer obstacles than before.

As Flo and JoAnn continued their walk around the unit, they passed the nurses' station and decided to peek inside. To their surprise, the huge wall clock—the one that had been as large as the wall itself—had shrunk to almost normal size. And the super-loud ticking of the clock was now a softer, more pleasant rhythm that was barely audible above the cheerful, animated conversations of the staff.

Off to the side, Mrs. Estello and her computer were humming in harmony. JoAnn leaned forward toward Mrs. Estello to see if she could recognize the tune. Almost immediately, a big smile spread across JoAnn's face.

She turned to Flo and whispered, "Listen! Mrs. Estello is humming 'Whistle While You Work'!"

"Maybe this *is* as good as it gets!" answered Flo. "Who would have thought that Mrs. Estello could ever be this happy about her job?"

As they walked away from the nurses' station, JoAnn and Flo heard some loud noises coming from outside. So they walked to a window they had never noticed before and peered out.

"What in the world . . . ?" began Flo.

"Well, I'll be. . . ." muttered JoAnn.

"It's another maze on another turf-covered field," said Flo. "And look—the maze is different from the one we saw on the field outside Radiology."

Indeed, Flo was right. This field was larger, and the

maze that dominated it was trickier than any of the great European castle garden mazes.

As Flo and JoAnn watched, they noticed that nurses, doctors, aides, and volunteers were moving patients along the maze. There were a few signs to guide the way, and some of the patients had maps that covered part of the maze. But there was still a lot of confusion, which caused many patients to get lost or go into dead ends.

From the ground level, the maze was puzzling and frustrating. Looking down from above, JoAnn and Flo could see that there was a much more direct route that would have been easier and faster for the hospital staff and their patients.

"Do you see what's happening?" Flo asked JoAnn.

"Yes," said JoAnn. "The Med-Surg team is racing through the maze, trying to get the patients to the end. They're moving very fast and working very hard. But they're making a lot of wrong moves."

"Right," said Flo. "I wish we could help them."

"Maybe we can," said JoAnn.

Just then, as the two women watched from the window, they noticed two nurses scaling one of the walls that surrounded the field. It was a tall, stone wall that seemed to reach up to the sky. But the climbers kept at it, slowly and steadily, finally reaching the top.

JoAnn and Flo watched as several other hospital employees, all dressed in green, applauded their success from down below. And then, suddenly, the climbers headed down the other side of the wall, disappearing from view.

"What do you think that was all about?" asked JoAnn.

"I don't know," answered Flo, just as confused as JoAnn.

"Well, I've seen enough," announced JoAnn. "I'm ready to head back to the normal world. I have an idea about how we might get those Zappometer readings higher than ever before!"

30

Back in the normal world of Med–Surg, JoAnn could hardly wait to get her staff together. She wanted to share what she'd learned by watching all of them from the 12th Dimension.

In no time, she'd collected her thoughts and called a unit meeting, inviting—as she had been doing for some time now—interested doctors and volunteers.

JoAnn was so excited that it would have been easy for her to jump right in with her idea. But instead, she wisely remembered to use the key principles as she addressed the group.

"Thanks so much for taking the time to be here for this important meeting," began JoAnn. "I especially appreciate the fact that Dr. Lee and Dr. Clayton could join us today."

JoAnn continued: "I am very proud of all the improvements you've been making through your participation on our Zapp! Teams. The patients are getting the best care ever, and we all seem happier about our jobs, and we have made definite improvements in holding down costs."

"That's right," said a number of people.

Then JoAnn asked, "Are we satisfied? Are we all doing the best we can?"

Considerable discussion followed, and everyone agreed that they could do more. To do more, though, they would have to attack the big problems facing the unit.

"I was thinking that it's as if our patients are moving through a *maze*," said JoAnn. "We have been working at ways to help them find their way through the maze and move faster, when maybe we should be asking the question, 'Does the maze have to be there in the first place?' "

"You're right," said Larry. "In fact, patients often refer to the hospital as a maze because it is so difficult to get anywhere. The processes they have to follow seem to make every task complicated."

Several others agreed that they needed to look for ways to improve the main processes in the Med–Surg unit.

"We need to find the fastest and most efficient path possible," added Flo.

"What I was hoping we could do today," continued JoAnn, "is to look for ways to improve and simplify our processes so we aren't running our patients all over the place unnecessarily."

And with that, she started to put in place the insight she had had while watching the unit from the 12th Dimension. She recorded it in her notebook.

JoAnn Mode's Notebook

It isn't enough to Zapp! people. We also have to *heal our processes!*

Zapped People
+ Improved Processes
Top Performance

"The first thing we need to do is to find out which processes need improvement," said JoAnn. "We have a lot of processes that are fine the way they are. We need to find the areas where improvement will have the greatest payoff."

Walking to a flip chart and picking up a marker, she said, "Let's make a list of all our processes, and then we will choose the ones where improvement would most impact our key result areas."

It took two meetings, but the team accomplished their task. First, they identified 25 different processes. Then, they determined the impact of each process on the unit's key result areas. Five critical processes emerged. The team decided to tackle the top two processes first and established a process improvement team for each: preoperative workup and bed availability.

It took a lot of practice, but in time Med-Surg was clearly streamlining its processes. And the unit discovered that improving the processes was resulting in other benefits as well.

For example, the staff found that they were happier doing their jobs because they weren't wasting time on unnecessary procedures and handoffs. They were also happy because the simplified processes allowed them more time for direct patient care.

Interestingly, Med-Surg also found that having simpler processes meant fewer errors, thus eliminating waste and rework. Through process improvement, JoAnn's unit had found ways to "do it right the first time."

Simpler processes also meant that the cost of caring for patients was lower. Because the processes were more efficient, the unit was hiring fewer temps and paying less overtime.

Perhaps the most obvious result of process improvement was that routine work activities really were simpler. Med-Surg had succeeded at simplifying procedures and employees' jobs.

And finally, JoAnn and her group were pleased to see that process improvements were allowing them to control the processes—not vice versa. By managing the processes, Med-Surg could better manage relationships with external suppliers and internal customers and ensure that suppliers' and customers' needs were met in the fastest, most efficient way possible.

JoAnn made sure she captured these discoveries in her notebook.

JoAnn Mode's Notebook

The benefits of process improvement:

- Employees are happier.
- Our customers—the patients—are happier, too.
- We eliminate errors.
- We simplify work activities.
- We control the processes instead of the processes controlling us.
- We lower the costs of patient care.

31

Little by little, the Med–Surg process improvement teams made progress. One of the things that helped them was to make a "map" of whatever process they wanted to improve. The teams would draw a map of the processes, tape the maps on the wall so everyone could see all the steps, and then look for areas to improve.

One team's surgeon member, Dr. Clayton, really got involved with *process mapping*. In fact, she did some research and showed the team that on their maps, certain symbols could represent various steps in the processes they were examining.

For example, a rectangle represented an activity step. A circle, an inspection step. A diamond, a decision step. An arrow represented process flow. A large "D," a delay. And an oval, the start or end of a process.

The team also decided to add a new symbol: a

big, black hole. This represented a point in the process where information goes in, but nothing comes out.

JoAnn made sure she put all these symbols in her notebook so she wouldn't forget them.

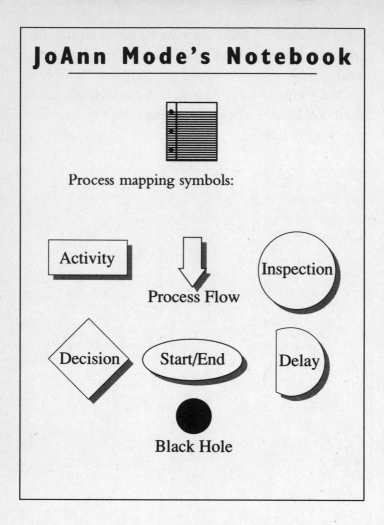

JoAnn Mode's Notebook

Process mapping symbols:

Activity

Process Flow

Inspection

Decision

Start/End

Delay

Black Hole

The maps made it easier for the group to see exactly what was happening at each step in the process. Once the team became familiar with the process mapping symbols, their maps really came alive.

The first thing they did with each process map was to simplify it. For example, the team decided to try to simplify the unit's process for handling doctors' orders for respiratory therapy as well as the actual delivery of the respiratory therapy. The original flow chart was pretty complicated.

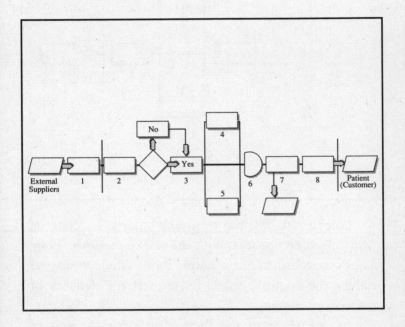

The simplified flow chart was, well, simpler.

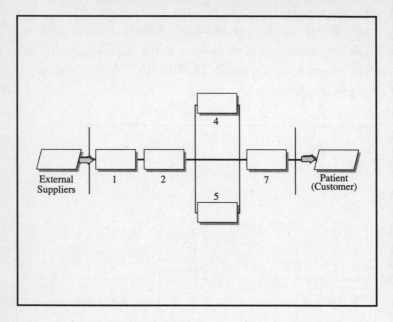

Needless to say, the team was anxious to share its new, improved process with the rest of the unit. They knew they had found a faster, more efficient way to handle the doctors' orders for request and delivery of respiratory therapy.

So the team shared their ideas with the rest of Med-Surg at the next staff meeting. JoAnn was especially happy when Dr. Clayton offered to be the team's spokesperson.

At the meeting, JoAnn watched as Dr. Clayton walked the group through the steps the team had taken. She explained everything clearly and then concluded her presentation by saying, "I'm convinced this process will work. It should help all of us do our jobs better and faster."

And Dr. Clayton was right: The new, simplified process was an improvement, and it did work. In fact, it worked so well that JoAnn heard Dr. Marcus telling Dr. Clayton one day, "You know, I used to order everything STAT from Respiratory Therapy because things took so long around here. I figured nobody would hurry unless they thought it was an emergency. But now I don't have to order everything STAT. Because the new processes work, I get what I need on time."

"Wow!" thought JoAnn. "Now we have people *and* processes that work! We're really on our way!"

JoAnn wrote in her notebook.

JoAnn Mode's Notebook

Process improvement steps:

1. Define the process boundaries—where a process starts and where it ends.
2. Identify your customers and suppliers.
3. Identify your customers' and suppliers' requirements.
4. Pinpoint the obstacles in your process path.
5. Develop an improvement plan to control or eliminate the major obstacles.

And remember: Every unit in a hospital has different processes. Every unit must find its own way.

About this time, JoAnn was feeling pretty smug about things when something happened to make her realize that *all* the hurdles weren't in the 12th Dimension.

32

One of Med-Surg's process improvement teams had been organized to tackle the long waiting times for the patients who needed lab tests, x-rays, and other services outside Med-Surg. Following the Action Cycle model, the team assessed the situation, determined causes, and targeted solutions and ideas. But when it came to implementing actions, they were stuck. So they went to their unit leader, JoAnn.

"How can we fix what's wrong when it involves other units?" the team wondered.

"That's a good question," said JoAnn. "I don't have an answer, but let me think about it."

To herself, JoAnn thought, "I think it's time for another trip to the 12th Dimension."

JoAnn asked Flo to join her, and off they went.

As soon as JoAnn Mode and Flo Knight got to the 12th Dimension, they headed for the field outside the Med-Surg unit. Right away, they could see that things were different—very different.

The maze, which had baffled and confused people

before, was now much easier. It now actually helped people get directly from one part of the field to the other.

"*Everyone* seems happier," said JoAnn.

Just then, the two women saw that off to the right, a tall ladder was being leaned against one of the high stone walls that surrounded the field.

"Now what?" thought JoAnn out loud.

"Some of the patients are using a ladder to climb over the walls," explained Flo. "It must be a shortcut to another unit."

"You mean there are other units and other mazes on the other side of the walls?" asked JoAnn.

"Yes," answered Flo. "Don't you remember when we were looking at the entire medical center from the 12th Dimension, and saw that *every* unit had a maze with walls separating one unit's maze from another. There are doors through the walls, but they don't seem to be in very convenient places."

"But why would all the hospital units have walls around them?" asked JoAnn "We all work *together*."

Flo was silent.

"Well, don't we?" asked JoAnn, pushing for an answer that she wasn't sure she wanted to hear.

"In some ways we work together," conceded Flo. "We're all trying to do the best we can for our patients. But many times the walls get in our way."

"What do you mean?" asked JoAnn.

"Remember when we noticed that the Radiology team's field, and our field, too, was covered with turf?"

"Yes," answered JoAnn.

"Well," explained Flo. "As I looked around the other day, I saw that *all* the fields were covered with turf."

"So?" asked JoAnn.

"We're showing all the symptoms of *turf-itis,*" began Flo.

"What?!"

"Turf-itis," repeated Flo. "It's a serious condition, and it's keeping all of us from giving our patients the very best care possible."

"I still don't understand," said JoAnn. "What in the world is turf-itis?"

"It's the *we-they* thinking that we're all prone to have," explained Flo. "You know, the *us-against-them* attitude we're all guilty of."

"But we're a *team* in Med-Surg!" said JoAnn. "There's no *we* or *they.*"

"What about outside Med-Surg?" asked Flo.

"We get along with people outside our own unit," said JoAnn. Then she added, "Well, most of the time."

"But sometimes we don't act like much of a *hospital team,*" said Flo. "Sometimes when our patients complain about waiting too long for lab results or x-rays, we blame the other departments for the delays instead of working together to improve the processes."

"You're right," admitted JoAnn.

"And our process improvement team usually looks only at improving things in our own unit," explained Flo. "When they tried to fix the problem of patients having to wait too long to get to Radiology or the lab? We got stuck because we don't know how to be partners with the other units. . . ."

JoAnn knew that Flo was right. She'd been feeling very proud of Med-Surg's accomplishments and, if she were honest about it, hadn't really *wanted* to share her ideas with the rest of the medical center.

JoAnn had to admit that she liked being a "star" and having one of the best-run units in the hospital.

But JoAnn also had to admit that Flo was right: If Normal Medical Center was going to provide the best possible care for its patients, then all those walls had to come down.

As JoAnn and Flo walked away, they decided to see what was happening in the Med-Surg hallways.

Not surprisingly, things were much less frantic than before. People moved about freely and easily, and they were walking briskly—not racing about wildly like before. Instead of the 12 hurdles that had been there before, there were only five. Improving Med-Surg's processes had made a big difference for everyone—not just the patients.

Just as Flo and JoAnn were commenting on how much better the unit looked, a huge gust of wind blew its way down the hallway, almost knocking them off their feet.

"What was that?" gasped JoAnn.

"I haven't a clue!" answered Flo, trying to catch her breath.

"Look!" said JoAnn. "Over there!"

As Flo turned to look in the direction JoAnn was pointing, she saw that the wind had blown in *hundreds* of pieces of paper. As the papers flew randomly throughout the halls, the Med–Surg doctors, nurses, and aides carried on with their tasks as usual. It seemed to Flo and JoAnn that nobody but them was paying any attention to the papers blowing here and there, hither and yon.

As the two women continued watching in amazement, the papers blew *everywhere*. Some of the papers landed in the hallway, right in the path of the doctors and staff. Some of the papers blew out the open windows and doorways, continuing on to other units and landing just as randomly as they had in Med–Surg. And some of the papers ended up in a huge pile in the corner by the nurses' station.

"What's going on?" asked JoAnn, still confused.

"It seems we still have a problem with paper," answered Flo. "There isn't as much as we had before, but it seems to be blowing in from the other units. Some of it stays here, and some of it just passes through on its way to other departments."

"I think you're right," said JoAnn. "What do you think that huge stack of papers is over there by the nurses' station?"

"I'm not sure," answered Flo. "But it looks like a fire hazard."

Flo had spoken not a moment too soon. As she and JoAnn looked on, they saw the familiar face of the dragon, peeking around the corner of the nurses' station. Spying the huge pile of papers, it smiled a wicked smile and spit a ball of fire on it. As the papers went up in flames, the dragon's smile grew even wider.

Of course, by now, Med–Surg was well prepared to deal with occasional fires on the unit, and everyone pitched in to dowse the flames with buckets of water. The dragon's smile slowly faded, and it made its way down the hallway, following the trail of papers that was making its way onto the other units. JoAnn and Flo could only wonder where—or when—the next fire would occur in Normal Medical Center.

"It looks as if we'll never really solve our paper problems—or any other problems—unless we work together with the other units," said JoAnn. "We need some *hospital-wide* process improvement teams, not just unit teams, because our processes are *interdependent*."

"I think we've discovered something important," said Flo. "We all have to work together to Zapp! Normal Medical Center."

And that's the discovery JoAnn and Flo took back to the three-dimensional world.

JoAnn wrote in her notebook.

JoAnn Mode's Notebook

To make major quality improvements, many parts of the hospital need to be involved—because all the units are interdependent.

PART V

Zapping the Medical Center

33

Though she could be quite trollish from time to time, Mary Ellen Krabofski was no dummy. In fact, she was very smart. She had been noticing that she had to spend very little time solving problems for Med-Surg or the Radiology department.

Of course, she knew about some amazing things going on in those units, such as the award Radiology had won. And she especially wanted to know why Med-Surg, where performance had always been mediocre at best, was now so great.

In fact, word had been spreading quickly throughout Normal Medical Center. Lots of nurses and aides wanted to transfer into these two units because both had earned the reputation of being wonderful places to work. Even some of the other unit supervisors had begun to ask what was going so *right* in Med-Surg and Radiology.

So when JoAnn and Claire asked for an opportunity to tell management about what they had been doing, Mary Ellen thought it was a good idea and set things up.

JoAnn and Claire went to their Zapp! Teams and asked for their help in developing a presentation for senior management. The teams went right to work.

First, they asked some radiologists and nurses to be part of the presentation, along with some physicians, aides, technologists, and volunteers. Then they started to plan who would do what. As the big day approached, JoAnn and Claire coached the Zapp! Team presenters on what to expect, what would be expected of them, and how to make a successful presentation.

When the big day arrived, JoAnn opened the presentation. She began by giving a glowing description of the power of Zapp! and how fantastic it was. Of course, no superlative for Zapp! was too great. Everyone was impressed.

Then she said, "Mary Ellen, we've wired your chair to the Flo-Vision. We're going to turn it on now, and in a moment you'll be whisked to the 12th Dimension where you'll see the wonders of Zapp! at work right before your very eyes."

JoAnn turned to the back of the room and said, "OK, Flo, hit it."

There was a high-pitched whine. Followed by a low-pitched whine. And then *nothing* happened.

"Excuse me. We seem to have some technical difficulties," muttered JoAnn.

With a reddened face, Flo stood up in the rear of

the room and said quietly, "Bad news, JoAnn, the Flo-Vision is broken. It blew its hootenannies."

JoAnn turned and looked at Mary Ellen.

The somewhat cross-eyed expression on Mary Ellen's face said it all: She was embarrassed.

Lightning, huh? Human lightning, you say? Yeah, right. *Wheels* of lightning, no less. Sure. Was there a *truck* attached to the wheels? Did you happen to get its license number?

Who could believe such nonsense?

Well, JoAnn made a very quick—and wise—decision. She continued with the presentation. The Zapp! Teams came up one by one. They talked about their accomplishments and how it felt to be Zapped. They talked about quality patient care, helping families, enhanced relationships with each other, and more efficient processes. They had tangible evidence of cost savings.

Dr. Clayton gave a fine testimonial about the power of Zapp! in Med-Surg, and then she offered rave reviews of the accomplishments of two of the process improvement teams. She even showed some of the unit's process maps.

"It's utterly amazing," added Dr. Marcus in his usual animated way. "Before Zapp!, everyone just did their jobs. But now we're having a *field day!*"

"Most important," he continued, "the doctors and hospital staff are working more closely together. And we're providing even better patient care than before at lower costs. More and more, I'm referring my patients to Normal Medical Center."

All these comments were magical music to senior management's ears.

And the *way* the Zapp! Team members talked demonstrated that Med-Surg and Radiology staff employees could take responsibility for their work on an everyday basis to a degree that people like Mary Ellen never would have thought possible.

As it turned out, they didn't need the Flo-Vision or the 12th Dimension to convince senior management. Best of all, Jerry Browning, the C.O.O., and Mary Ellen Krabofski were impressed. By the end of the presentation, they were positively Zapped!

Mary Ellen wanted her other units to be Zapped the same way—right away.

"We have to tell everyone about this!" exclaimed Mary Ellen. She was very excited. "I want every unit to have teams—uh, what are you calling them? Zapp! Teams? That's it, *Zapp! Teams!* I want all our units to start using Zapp! ASAP!"

No one is more dedicated to a cause than a skeptic who becomes convinced.

The very next day, Mary Ellen scheduled a meeting of all the unit supervisors, attempting to convince them that Zapp! was the way for everybody to go.

This didn't work.

The other supervisors nodded their heads, agreed that Zapp! made sense, and then went back to being the same kind of supervisors they had always been.

But from this, Mary Ellen learned something important.

To create Zapp!, she had to use Zapp!

The other hospital units had to discover Zapp! on their own. With her enZapping help, of course.

She began with the three principles of Zapp!

1. **Maintain or enhance self-esteem.**
2. **Listen and respond with empathy.**
3. **Ask for help and encourage involvement.**

Mary Ellen began practicing these principles when dealing with administrative peers, nurses, aides, technologists, support personnel, and anyone else she happened to run into. And, of course, she found that the principles were as applicable to her as they were to JoAnn, Claire, or anyone else in a leadership role.

Then she applied the soul of Zapp!:

**Offer help without
taking responsibility for action.**

One day, the Emergency department supervisor called Mary Ellen about a problem involving her unit. Normally, Mary Ellen would have headed up an investigation and put herself in charge. But this time she asked the unit supervisor what should be done and then offered her help in implementing the plan. She coached and added input from her own experience, but the problem and the solution clearly remained with the Emergency department.

Zapp!

As the director of nursing, Mary Ellen realized that she had an essential role to play: to support the kind of environment where Zapp! could develop and flourish.

For instance, she encouraged all the unit supervisors to get formal training in Zapp!, and she made available the resources for this training to take place.

Then, just as JoAnn had done for Med-Surg, Mary Ellen asked all the other unit supervisors to develop performance guidelines with key result areas, measurements, and goals.

Mary Ellen also found that she had some changes to make with her own staff.

Flo, JoAnn, and Claire reported that just when a wheel of Zapp! was turning its fastest and shining its brightest, some source of Sapp¡ often would come along to dull it.

Some of these Sapps were BIG ONES.

Big enough even to bring the wheels almost to a stop.

For instance, Claire told Mary Ellen about something that had happened just last week.

Hugh Lancelot (wearing a normal business suit instead of his 12th Dimension shining armor) had walked unexpectedly into the Radiology department and announced that he and his associates were going to assess the unit based on new federal standards.

"What makes this evaluation different from the one we had last fall?" Claire had asked.

"We have changed the standards," said Hugh. "It's pretty philosophical, so you wouldn't understand. All you need to know is that we have all the answers. We'll take care of everything. We are here to help you."

Sapp¡

"Mr. Lancelot, how can I help?" asked Claire.

"No need. We will do it all," was the reply. "We will assess your department and write a report on our findings," he explained, holding up an evaluation booklet that was at least three inches thick. "If you want a copy, write to us in three months."

Based on the way Hugh and his crew were acting, Claire knew that this process would be a big Sapp¡ for her department. She tried to explain about the Zapp! Teams and suggested getting the appropriate team members involved. She knew that there wcrc cnZapping ways to handle an assessment, so she pleaded with him to listen.

But Hugh Lancelot was set in his ways, and he had his orders from on high. Once he began his work, there was nothing Claire could do about it.

Hugh Lancelot and his associates treated the staff objectively—that is, like objects. They hurriedly visited every area in the department with their three-inch-thick booklet and said very little to the technologists. They just took note after note.

"What did you think?" asked Claire proudly, as Hugh and his team started out the door.

"Can't reveal my findings—they're top secret. But I can tell you this. Most of your technologists are not following the recommended procedures. Your staff has too much freedom. You should be spending more time supervising and less time promoting your so-called teams," said Hugh.

Sapp¡¡

JoAnn had been on her way to see Mary Ellen about some supplies she needed for Med-Surg when she was intercepted by a man in the hallway outside her office.

"Hello, I'm Biff Buffer, the new assistant to the director of nursing," he said. "Talk to me when you need anything from now on."

JoAnn explained her request, and Biff said, "Hmm. I can't give you the go-ahead on something like that right now. You know money is tight. I'll have to clear that with M.E. the next time I see her, and of course I'll have to talk with the C.O.O. to see if funds are available. Check back with me in about three or four weeks, and maybe I'll have a decision by then."

"Three or four weeks?" asked JoAnn, not quite believing her ears.

"Weeks? Did I say *weeks?* Oh, sorry. I meant three or four *months.*"

Sapp¡¡¡

"Oh," said Mary Ellen to Claire, JoAnn, and Flo. "I guess we need to make some changes. We have to check our systems and regulations to see if they are aligned with Zapp!—and obviously my staff needs some training, too. Thanks."

To be quite honest, it took Mary Ellen a long time to relinquish the keys to the executive fire truck. It wasn't easy. But as she continued to apply Zapp!, a change came over her.

In fact, when JoAnn took her occasional walks around the 12th Dimension, she hardly recognized Mary Ellen. Her color was no longer ghastly green. Her scales had melted. Her tail grew shorter, and then it disappeared. Soon, she was no longer a troll. Zapp! had changed her into a human being, the true form of all good directors of nursing.

When JoAnn talked with Mary Ellen about the changes, they talked about what they had learned. And JoAnn made sure she wrote everything down so that she wouldn't forget.

JoAnn Mode's Notebook

Senior management's role in spreading Zapp!:

- To ensure that everyone in the organization has the interpersonal, team, and problem-solving skills needed to implement Zapp! (If necessary, provide more training.)
- To promote people to leadership positions who are motivated to Zapp! others.
- To be sure that unit leaders and team leaders have the skills required to Zapp! (And if they don't, get them into training.)
- To coach supervisors and their staffs on how to use and improve their Zapp! skills.
- To reward performance resulting from Zapp!

Notebook 📓 (cont'd)

- To ensure that systems, policies, and regulations reinforce Zapp! and that the people in charge of these systems, policies, and regulations have the necessary Zapp! skills.

Overall: To create an environment where Zapp! can happen.

Management was trying hard, but things weren't always simple. Providing training, for example, was a lot harder than they imagined.

34

Now you'd think that training in Zapp! skills would be a natural for a hospital *filled* with highly trained people. But alas, it was not that easy.

A team was formed to define what needed to be taught to whom, and JoAnn and Claire were asked to join. It was decided that everyone, at all levels, should have the same basic skills so they could work well with one another. JoAnn's experience in developing the skills of people on her unit was helpful in determining what these basic skills were. After discussion by the team, JoAnn revised a page in her notebook.

JoAnn Mode's Notebook

Basic Zapp! skills (revised):

• People skills for interacting with one another. (Stress the key principles.)
• Meeting membership and leadership skills.
• Problem solving and idea implementation skills. (Stress the Action Cycle.)
• Process identification and improvement.

These skills are important at all levels.

The method of training people in these skills may be different for different levels.

Additional discussion and a survey of the most effective leaders in the medical center helped to define unique leader needs. These discoveries were dutifully recorded in JoAnn's notebook, too.

JoAnn Mode's Notebook

Unit leaders need training on how to promote quality and excellence in patient care through Zapp!

Specifically, hospital unit leaders need training on how to:

- Effectively delegate and set up procedures to monitor what's going on in their units.
- Help individual employees establish performance expectations, recognizing that people and situations differ.
- Coach and reinforce employees on achieving goals.
- Encourage and support initiative.
- Promote teamwork within and among units.

Notebook 📓 (cont'd)

- Encourage and reinforce efforts aimed at continuous improvement in patient care and service.
- Model use of patient interaction skills when called upon, particularly in high-stress situations.

Note: Remember to use the key principles!

Mary Ellen was very happy with the lists. Then she realized that these were the same leadership skills needed to meet the Joint Commission's mandates *and* ensure that employees' actions supported quality objectives. This made her even happier.

Developing skills was a lot harder!

First, the employees were placed into classes where they heard lectures about Zapp! People didn't change much.

Next, Mary Ellen tried role-playing. Selected trainees were called to the front of the room and told to imagine that they were in a difficult situation where they had the opportunity to use Zapp! Then they were asked to demonstrate what they would do. Most would fail, and then their failures would be discussed by the class, as the instructor made learning points based on the roleplayers' mistakes.

Few skills were learned, because only a few people actually got to practice. And the roleplayers lost confidence in themselves because of their failure experiences. Seeing what had happened to the roleplayers, the rest of the class realized that they would also find it difficult if placed in a similar situation in real life, and their confidence went down, too.

Then, there was the problem of time. Everyone thought skill training was a good idea, but nobody wanted to spend the time to do it.

Several of the unit supervisors attended an outside course, where they spent three days learning Zapp! skills. Based on their glowing report, the hospital's administration decided to hold an in-house program. However, the hospital allowed only one day for what had been covered by the experts in three days. Not surprisingly, it didn't have the same impact.

Observing all this, JoAnn got out her notebook and wrote down some of what she'd learned about behavioral skills training.

JoAnn Mode's Notebook

Behavioral skills training:

- It's hard to preach people into changing their behavior.
- Developing confidence is just as important as developing skills.
- Changing behavior takes time. There is no substitute for practice with feedback. Watching someone else practice doesn't do it.

Much to its credit, Normal Medical Center continued to experiment. After one particularly frustrating training experience, one of the Pediatrics nurses made the comment, "It seems that what we've learned about coaching patients could help us in our training programs. When I worked last week with Mindy, for example, a young patient just diagnosed with diabetes, I started off by checking to be sure she understood the long-term importance of a stable blood sugar level.

Next, we talked about how the insulin would help her stabilize her blood sugar level, and I explained how to give injections. Then I showed her what to do and helped her practice."

"The practice is what's missing from our training programs," continued the nurse. "We need to work in smaller groups and be able to practice."

"Oh, no. We couldn't do that," said a senior manager. "Imagine how much it would cost to give everybody an opportunity to practice the skills in every training program."

But after much discussion, they settled the issue with a telling insight: *Any money spent on training that doesn't work is wasted. No matter how cheap or short the training is.*

And so senior management looked into more effective options. At first, changing from a lecture format was a difficult transition for the hospital administrators and employees. Most everyone's past training had involved lecture/discussion formats, with a few case studies or other exercises thrown in. Anything else seemed strange.

After a little investigation, though, Mary Ellen found that the technology they were exploring had a name: *behavior modeling*. She also found that a great deal of research had been done about its effectiveness in developing people's skills and confidence.

Mary Ellen shared this information with all the unit leaders (as they were now called), and that's how it got into JoAnn's notebook.

JoAnn Mode's Notebook

Behavior modeling is a classroom application of coaching that is effective in training staff and leaders. Behavior modeling steps:

1. Discuss the importance and relevance of the skill to be learned.
2. Discuss the principles or steps important to becoming successful in the skill.
3. Demonstrate the principles or steps. (Consider using videotape demonstrations.)
4. Allow each participant an opportunity to practice the new skill and to receive feedback.
5. Coach participants prior to their practice opportunity to ensure success.

Notebook (cont'd)

6. Train the participants who are observing the skill practice session to give supportive, balanced feedback.

7. Before they leave the training session, encourage the participants to commit to specific on-the-job applications.

At least five skill practice sessions are necessary for the average participant to develop skills and confidence in using the Zapp! key principles.

Unit leaders need to be trained in the same skills as the staff. In addition, they need to know how to coach and reinforce employees' on-the-job application of the skills learned.

JoAnn learned from Mary Ellen that the thing that made behavior modeling training in Zapp! skills effective was that after people had a success in trying out skills in the nurturing environment of a training room, they had the confidence to use the skills on the job.

On-the-job successes of the employees who had been trained, combined with supportive reinforcement from their supervisors and coworkers, created even more confidence. So they kept becoming more skilled and more confident.

It wasn't easy, and it certainly didn't work all the time. But behavior modeling got the right skills into the hands of the right people, and that's what everyone wanted.

35

As more employees were trained in the skills necessary to be Zapped, and as leaders learned how to Zapp!, teams started to pop up all over Normal Medical Center. Some teams tackled unit problems that affected service efficiency, like delays in responding to equipment repair work orders, supply shortages, Housekeeping response time, and effectiveness in the O.R.s.

Attacking bigger cross-unit or total medical center issues became the responsibility of cross-unit or cross-functional teams. Some of the teams were made up of nurses, like the team formed to investigate continuing education courses available at Normal Nursing College.

Other teams crossed positions, like the Staff Recognition Team, which included all interested staff, doctors, and volunteers. This team looked for ways to recognize and reward exceptional performance throughout the hospital.

Another team decided to apply for the honor of being named a Hospital of Excellence by the Universal

Hospital Foundation. "How about that," thought JoAnn, "from normal to excellent. I like that!"

Still another team decided that in order to promote professionalism throughout Normal Medical Center, they would create a small resource center on the unit. The team's goal was not only to house the latest professional journals and literature in the center, but to create an environment conducive to professional development: a place where employees could catch up on information about the latest standards of care, new equipment, etc. The hospital's volunteers helped by holding a used-book sale in order to raise funds for the team, which had its own budget and was responsible for selecting all its own materials.

To JoAnn's surprise, even Mrs. Estello got into the act. After she saw the success of other teams, she decided that the clerks could work on solving problems, too.

So she called a friend of hers who was a clerk in Pediatrics, and then the two of them recruited half a dozen other clerks at Normal Medical Center. At their first meeting, they decided to tackle the issue of a dress code for office workers throughout the hospital. They had noticed an increasing problem of some employees dressing inappropriately, particularly in Admissions, the Business Office, and other areas where employees interacted with the public.

The clerical team surveyed another hospital and several businesses. After completing their surveys, they drafted a dress code that they believed would help the hospital present a more positive image. Then they presented it to senior management, with JoAnn and Mary Ellen's complete support.

The dress code, which was heartily approved by Normal Medical Center's senior management, was distributed to all employees and, eventually, incorporated into the handbooks given to new personnel. Needless to say, JoAnn was very proud of Mrs. Estello's initiative. And Mrs. Estello was proud, too.

Identifying major opportunities became the focus of hospital-wide process improvement teams. For example, one team was able to reduce the time it took to admit patients from 40 minutes to 10 minutes. Another team reduced bed availability delays by 50 percent. Even the doctors got involved, reducing lengths of stay for the top four volume D.R.G.s by 25 percent.

Not that all the Zapp! Teams worked perfectly. Some got off track. Some didn't feel a real management commitment to their tasks. And others developed interpersonal or interunit rivalries or other problems. Sometimes, intervention by a leader would get the team back on track, through coaching and clarification of roles and expectations. Sometimes, refresher training did the trick. A few times, nothing worked, and teams had to be disbanded—to be reconstructed at another time.

As management developed more confidence in the hospital teams, they decided to create a team with representatives from each hospital unit to tackle the difficult task of recommending a major reorganization.

This was a real challenge: to find ways to restructure Normal Medical Center so that it could provide even better services in timely, cost-effective ways.

This team, affectionately known around the hospital as "Wallbusters," was intent on coming up with creative solutions for an age-old problem: knocking down the "walls" that existed between units. The team knew that for the hospital to operate as one large team, these barriers had to be removed.

But how?

Well, first the team called in all the Zapp! experts—JoAnn, Flo, Claire, and Mary Ellen—for advice on interunit walls. They were all asked to join the team.

Second, they made sure they had senior management's support. They knew this would be essential for the success of any hospital reorganization efforts.

Third, they researched what other hospitals were doing around the country. What was working? What wasn't? What were the costs of reorganizing?

Fourth, they *asked for help* from Normal Medical Center's own doctors and staff. What did *they* think their patients needed?

And finally, they asked their patients for ideas.

Right away, the reorganization team found that their assignment was a challenging one. Almost everyone, it seemed, thought that because hospitals had always been organized into separate units, that was the only way it *could* be.

"This is a huge shift in thinking," JoAnn said to Flo

one day. "It's as if a lot of us *like* our walls. They give us structure and security."

"You're right, JoAnn," said Flo. "But as you've always said, we have to keep looking for better ways."

Assembling all their information, the team talked.

And talked.

And talked some more.

Finally, using all their new problem-solving and process improvement skills, they came up with a plan to present to senior management. They were sure it was a good plan.

The team expected their leader to make the presentation. But she had a better idea: "Why don't we *all* present our plan? After all, every member of the team has shared in the hard work. And we're all responsible for coming up with the new plan. We should *all* make the presentation."

"Great idea," said Flo.

Well, the big day came, and the team was ready.

Each team member handled a specific part of the presentation, and Mary Ellen summarized for the group.

"So," began Mary Ellen, "what we're recommending is to divide Normal Medical Center into five mini hospitals or 'patient care centers.' Each center would specialize in one area of medicine, and each would operate independently."

"With the new arrangement," continued Mary Ellen, "a group of about 10 to 12 patients would be placed in a geographically contained area that we would call a pod. The patients in each pod would be treated by a team of hospital employees who had been cross-trained in various tasks."

The room was silent.

"Oh-oh," thought Mary Ellen. "Something's wrong. This group *always* has something to say. Maybe I should repeat the main points of the proposal to be sure they understand."

But she remained silent because she knew if she did, it would have been a Sapp¡ for the team.

Finally, Jerry Browning spoke.

"I think this could work," said Jerry. "We will need to talk more about the implications for costs and cross-training, but you have developed a good plan. Thank you."

"Let's adjourn for today and meet again next week," continued the C.O.O. "Between now and then, we'll all be able to formulate questions, and from there we'll move on to determining what we need to turn your idea into reality."

"Wow!" thought JoAnn. "Even C.O.O.s can Zapp!"

36

By now, more and more doctors were referring their patients to Normal Medical Center. In fact, the patient load had grown so much that the existing nursing staff couldn't possibly do everything they needed to do to provide quality care for all their patients. Even with all the process improvements, the hospital needed more nurses.

One of the units that found itself short-staffed was Med-Surg. So, as she was obligated to do by Normal policy, JoAnn went to the Personnel department with the proper authorizations from Mary Ellen, and Personnel approved her hiring request.

A while later, Theresa showed up. A recent graduate of Normal Nursing College, this was her first job. "They sent me over. Guess I'm your new R.N.," said Theresa.

JoAnn introduced her to the Med-Surg staff. And the other nurses and aides took an instant dislike to Theresa.

It wasn't that there was anything *wrong* with Theresa. She was not a fugitive from justice or wanted by the FBI, and she had all the proper credentials for the position. But nobody could get very excited about having Theresa on the Med–Surg team.

Why should they? No one on the Med–Surg staff had been involved in selecting Theresa. Nothing was personally at stake for any of them if Theresa didn't work out.

Not even JoAnn Mode had a stake in Theresa's success. No one in the Personnel department had even asked JoAnn about the special requirements for a nurse on her unit.

And Theresa was not very excited about her new assignment either. Med–Surg? Big deal. *They* hadn't selected her. The *personnel director* had selected her.

Theresa was Sapped for a long time.

JoAnn realized this, and the next time Med–Surg needed a new nurse, she asked Mary Ellen to talk to the Personnel department about modifying the procedures in order to make them more enZapping.

Mary Ellen gladly presented the situation to the personnel director and asked for her help in working with JoAnn and the other unit leaders.

And this time, the results were very different.

The nurses developed a list of dimensional competencies needed for success in Med–Surg. They were careful to include technical, interpersonal, and problem-solving dimensions. Each was defined through on-the-job examples so that everyone understood them clearly.

Next, JoAnn and some of her nurses were trained in how to conduct behavior-based interviews targeted to the dimensions. Two nurses plus JoAnn interviewed each candidate.

They also devised creative ways to evaluate how well the candidates would fit into a Zapped unit. For example, candidates were given a standard description about a hypothetical patient with multiple health problems who was difficult to get along with. After time to prepare, each candidate conducted a simulated meeting with the "patient" (played by one of the nurses). Another nurse observed the simulated interaction and evaluated the candidate's interpersonal skills using special observation forms so that all candidates would be evaluated according to the same criteria.

After much discussion about the strengths and weaknesses of each candidate compared with the list of predetermined target dimensions, the nurses made a decision about which candidate to hire. It was a big Zapp! for everyone.

It was a Zapp! for the personnel director: She could see that the unit was getting a nurse who would be effective and comfortable in a Zapped environment.

It was a Zapp! for the Med-Surg staff because

the nurses had had a say in who would work with them. Taking part in the selection decision gave the nurses ownership in the selected nurse's success. They naturally took on responsibility for the individual's development and willingly did everything they could to ensure that the chosen nurse would be successful.

Involving nurses in the selection process also helped to develop the hiring nurses. This was because setting up and running the selection process had helped everyone involved become better nurses by encouraging them to focus on the specific behaviors really important to nursing success in Med-Surg.

Not surprisingly, it was a huge Zapp! for the new nurse to be chosen by the unit leader and the Med-Surg nursing team instead of being imposed upon them. In fact, the new nurse worked even harder than usual to keep from disappointing her new colleagues.

JoAnn wrote in her notebook.

JoAnn Mode's Notebook

- Selecting people with the right skills and the motivation to be Zapped saves a lot of training and coaching time.

- Selection need not be a "toss of the coin." Accuracy can be improved by focusing interviews on a list of predetermined job requirements.

- Using simulations of what candidates will face on the job provides important additional insights into specific skill areas.

37

One of the biggest surprises of all at Normal Medical Center was how good the *patients'* ideas were!

As the staff continued developing patient surveys, and as hospital employees and volunteers kept talking with patients about patient needs, they learned that the hospital's "customers" really knew what they wanted!

For example, one patient, whose eyesight was failing her, suggested asking the hospital's volunteers if they'd be willing to read to patients who, for whatever reason, couldn't read for themselves. Several volunteers jumped at the chance to provide this additional service, and they even went a step further: The volunteers started a small "lending library" of popular books and magazines that could be used by the volunteer readers as well as any interested patients or visitors. The lending library also included audiotapes and large-print books.

As the lending library's popularity grew, Normal's volunteers collected used books from the community, and they sponsored a bake sale to raise money for buying additional books and magazine subscriptions.

Another patient suggested that larger, more comfortable hospital gowns were long overdue—and he was right! A team was set up to investigate options. They followed the Action Cycle steps and came up with a cost-effective gown in a larger size.

The team was surprised to find that such a small change could have such a big impact on patient satisfaction. Almost as soon as the larger gowns were made available, patients began complimenting the hospital on the improvement. As one patient put it, "Now I can concentrate on getting better instead of worrying that my gown isn't covering everything it should!"

Another patient suggested a "buddy" system for pairing up Normal's patients with former patients who had recovered from similar types of surgery. The staff found this idea was especially well received by some of the oncology patients, who were encouraged by talking with a person who was in remission.

Yet another patient suggested an idea that did away with asking patients to fill out the same medical history checklists again and again as they moved from one unit to another. The patient thought it would be a good idea to treat patients like customers in a department store and open "accounts" for them when they first got to Normal. Using Normal Medical Center's new computer network, a process improvement team succeeded in finding a way to get pertinent information to every department that needed it, with the patient going through the medical history checklist only once.

One of Normal's outpatients suggested that the

medical center could meet patient needs better by creating an intermediate type of daytime care that would offer services somewhere between inpatient and outpatient care. Because outpatient surgeries were becoming more common, more people were finding themselves being treated as outpatients than ever before, and some needed more care than others. An intensive outpatient service for handling subacute care would allow the medical center to provide all-day care for those outpatients who needed it, and those outpatients who required less care could continue to receive outpatient services in the normal way.

When a team presented this idea to senior management, they had done their homework. Several members of the team had talked with other hospitals that offered intensive outpatient services and had found that a graduated fee schedule was used. If, for example, the daily rate was $500 for inpatients, then intensive outpatient care might cost $200 a day.

Senior management was impressed! They continued to Zapp! by empowering the team to implement their idea.

One of Normal's hearing-impaired patients suggested many good ideas. Kristin, who had lost most of her hearing at the age of three, offered to talk with interested hospital staff members about how they could help their hearing-impaired patients.

Coached by a team charged with improving patient care, Kristin explained that it was very important for health care providers to look at her directly when speaking, and not have their backs turned toward her; this way, she could read their lips. Kristin offered other tips, too: Be sure you have the patient's attention before you begin speaking, speak clearly at a moderate pace, use facial expressions and gestures, and be patient if the first try isn't successful.

As the team listened to Kristin's ideas, they began to realize how confusing—or even frightening—a hospital experience could be for a hearing-impaired patient. They also realized the need to have staff and volunteers on board who knew sign language, and they looked into starting an introductory sign language class at the hospital.

Kristin helped the team understand the importance of being sure a hearing-impaired patient understood exactly what was going to happen next, especially in a situation involving surgery or some other setting where the patient's hearing aids would have to be removed.

"And speaking of surgery," said Kristin, "I've read that some surgeons are now using clear masks instead of the usual cloth masks so that hearing-impaired patients can read the doctors' lips even after their hearing aids have been removed in the operating room."

As Kristin talked with team members, it was obvious that she was truly interested in helping other patients. So they asked Kristin if she'd be willing to serve on their team on a long-term basis. "I'd love to!" said Kristin, pleased to know that the team considered her ideas valuable.

After talking with Kristin, the team began to think

about other patients' special needs. What about interpreters for patients whose understanding of the English language was limited? And what about extra help for those patients who had trouble understanding the hospital's forms and instructions?

Family support groups also sprang up as a result of patients' ideas. They included monthly support groups for families of alcohol- and drug-dependent patients, diabetes patients, and cancer survivors.

Perhaps one of the most significant improvements to occur at Normal as a result of a patient's idea was the change in policy regarding a more liberal use of painkillers in the first hours and days after surgery. The patient, who had read about new federally supported guidelines for handling post-operative pain, suggested that Normal Medical Center consider alternatives to the traditional approach, which was to administer painkillers only at certain intervals and only when patients strongly requested relief.

A team representing nurses, surgeons, clinical pharmacists, and anesthesiologists was formed to look into options. One team member reviewed the federal guidelines and found that they urged greater use of alternatives to drugs, such as simple relaxation techniques, heat, cold packs, and massage. She also learned that the guidelines had been recommended by experts and tested in hospitals for their effectiveness.

The doctors on the team were optimistic about exploring ways to ease their patients' post-op pain, and they agreed to discuss the subject further with their colleagues.

Because of the nature of this change, going through the proper channels was important, and the team had to be patient. But in the end, Normal amended its policy about responding to patients' post-op pain to assure that a nurse coordinated the development of individualized pain control plans with patients and their doctors before surgery.

Now *that* was a Zapp!

An especially important team created a new brochure called "Patients' Rights and Responsibilities." While the idea of a patients' bill of rights had been around for a while, this brochure added a new twist: patients' *responsibilities*.

The recognition that patients have responsibilities as well as rights was important to the team because they knew that an important part of Zapp! was responsibility. If Normal patients were to receive the best care possible *and* be true members of the Normal Medical Center team, then they needed to accept certain responsibilities, too—just like all the other members of the Normal team.

The team was somewhat surprised at the enthusiastic response of the patients who were helping to develop the brochure on patients' rights and responsibilities. They had assumed that they would hear a lot of ideas about *rights* and very few ideas about *responsibilities*.

But the team was wrong.

Most of the patients recognized the importance of personal involvement in their treatment plans and offered good ideas for inclusion in the brochure.

For example, some of the patients' *rights* were:

- The right to be treated with respect by competent personnel.
- The right to high-quality care and high professional standards.
- The right to privacy, whenever possible.
- The right to confidentiality of all medical records and patient access to those records.
- The right to know Normal Medical Center's rules and regulations.
- The right to expect emergency procedures to be implemented without unnecessary delay.
- The right to full disclosure of information about the patient's diagnosis, treatment, and prognosis.
- The right to refuse any procedure, treatment, or drugs offered by Normal Medical Center.
- The right to obtain a second opinion.
- The right to receive all services without discrimination.
- The right to have time managed efficiently by Normal Medical Center in order to make effective use of the patient's time and to avoid personal discomfort.
- The right to receive a detailed explanation of the bill, along with information about any available financial resources.

- The right to a thorough explanation upon discharge of the patient's continuing medical requirements.

Some of the patients' *responsibilities* were:

- Providing accurate information about past illnesses, hospitalization, medication, etc., related to medical history.
- Cooperating with the staff in the treatment and recovery plans.
- Asking questions if directions or procedures are not clearly understood.
- Being considerate of other patients and staff regarding the control of noise, smoking, number of visitors, and care of hospital property.
- Following health care instructions.
- Accepting financial responsibility for all services rendered.
- Refraining from using any nonprescribed drugs or alcohol during the hospital stay.

After the "Patients' Rights and Responsibilities" brochure was completed, it became a standard handout for all patients. And whenever possible, the assigned nurses and aides gave the brochure to new patients in person, welcoming them to Normal Medical Center and assuring them that the staff would try to make their stays as pleasant as possible.

And that was always a Zapp!

By far, one of the most enjoyable parts of being a member of the teams involved in improving patient services was reading all the notes and cards that came into Normal Medical Center from former patients and their families. It seemed that the more Zapp! there was among health care providers, the more Zapp! was felt by the patients and their families.

It was decided that everyone in the hospital should have the opportunity to read these testimonials about the excellent care received at Normal Medical Center, so a large display area was set up in the main lobby where all incoming letters and cards could be posted.

One of the letters read:

Dear Friends,

You were all so wonderful during my recent stay at Normal Medical Center that I had to write and say thank you.

Everyone was very kind and always treated me with dignity. I felt as if my nurses and doctors were really taking care of me—not just doing their jobs. It was so nice to find that in this age of "high technology," the people at Normal Medical Center remember to use "high touch" and healthy doses of compassion.

The support staff was great, too. The dietician worked with me so I would understand my new diet and be able to manage on my own once I got home. And the pharmacist even helped me locate a drug store that will deliver my prescriptions right to my door.

When I was asked to fill out your patient survey questionnaire, I was stumped by the question, "What could we do to improve our services?" I say, JUST KEEP DOING WHAT YOU'RE DOING!

Thank you for everything.

> Sincerely,
> Beth Sommers

"Dear *Friends*. . . ." Everyone liked that.

38

Years passed.

One morning, JoAnn Mode was working in her office when Phyllis knocked on her door and said, "Excuse me, JoAnn, but there's a young woman out here who says she'd like to ask you some questions about how we run the Med–Surg unit."

JoAnn asked Phyllis to send her in.

"What's your name?" JoAnn asked the young woman, as she sat down.

"I'm Kate," said the young woman.

"Well, Kate, what can I do for you?"

"I'm the new unit supervisor in Pediatrics, and Mary Ellen Krabofski sent me over here to learn about something called Zapp! I understand your unit was one of the first to start using it," said Kate.

"That's true," said JoAnn proudly.

"I've heard that Zapp! is the energy that fosters continuous improvement."

"That's also true," said JoAnn.

"Well, how does it work?" asked Kate.

By now, JoAnn was quite accustomed to inquiries by the curious. She'd been explaining Zapp! to unit leaders and hospital employees for years. And it seemed that every month, she had something new to report.

As they talked, JoAnn took Kate for a tour, showing her the Med–Surg unit and introducing her to some of the Zapp! Teams, whose members gladly explained what they did and how they worked together. Most of the team members were careful to point out that learning about Zapp! took a lot of time and energy. It wasn't an easy process. But the results were definitely worth it.

At the end of the tour, JoAnn took Kate to the 12th Dimension so that she could see Zapp! in living color. Finally, to give Kate the big picture, JoAnn showed her a new feature of the 12th Dimension: It was a big, round observation deck that afforded a magnificent view of Normal Medical Center and other hospitals in the distance.

From horizon to horizon, through the gaps in the drifting mists and fog, they could see all kinds of hospital castles scattered about the countryside.

Over here, on a rocky rise, was a large castle, which looked much like the Normal Medical Center castle had years ago, with sentries posted and lots of people coming and going through its gates.

And over there was a crumbling, dark, deserted castle sinking into a swamp.

Off on the horizon was Typical Medical Center, a huge, high, and impossibly complex castle with towers reaching into the clouds—into and *above* the clouds, in fact. Its top administrators probably couldn't even see the ground from up there. With its miles of maze-like walls and moats, it looked like nothing could ever topple Typical, that it would stand forever.

But just then, gliding among the tallest towers, JoAnn and Kate saw *flying* dragons. As they watched, one of the dragons, clinging to the side of one of the biggest towers, munched its way through the walls—chomp, chomp, chomp—until the tower fell over like an axed tree and landed with an enormous crash. Indeed, for all its size and grim complexity, the Typical castle seemed hopelessly antiquated compared to the shape of their own Normal Medical Center.

In fact, most of Normal Medical Center these days did not even look like a castle. Normal Medical Center looked more like a launching pad, a home base for health care professionals who took off every morning in a wide-ranging fleet of amazing crafts that had been designed with the help of those who flew them. The fleet was propelled by the energy of Zapp!

As JoAnn and Kate looked around, they could see all the Normal Medical Center doctors, employees, and volunteers out there in the wild blue, flying their missions and caring for patients. Best of all, they were all piloting their own space crafts—many with fantastic shapes they had designed for specific patient needs.

Kate noticed that the Normal Medical Center launching pad was situated on a huge, sprawling field. JoAnn explained that long ago, the large field had been made up of many smaller fields that were separated by high, stone walls.

"In a few places," JoAnn pointed out, "we still have some walls, but they're much lower—so low that our hospital staff can step right over them as they move from one unit to another."

"Look!" said Kate. "Over there!"

As JoAnn looked on, a construction crew arrived in a bright yellow truck. On the side of the truck was printed "Wallbusters!" The crew, all wearing hard hats, carried huge sledgehammers. They went straight to one of the remaining walls and, with fierce determination, began tearing it down. The onlookers cheered.

"We're making real progress," JoAnn said to Kate. "Someday *all* the walls will be gone!

"We had a serious case of "*turf-itis,*" JoAnn continued. "It was almost an epidemic.

"But now," JoAnn said proudly, "everyone moves around Normal Medical Center freely from one area to another. We've realized that we're all on the same team.

"Our teams used to feel as if they were moving patients through a *maze,*" JoAnn continued. "But now it's more like a huge playing field. Look over there! Some of our patients are playing frisbee with the staff!"

"They're having so much *fun!*" said Kate. "Aren't they supposed to be working?"

"They *are* working," explained JoAnn. "But for every Normal Medical Center staff member, doctor, and volunteer, it feels *good* to go to work. Their ordinary jobs aren't ordinary any more."

"But don't we ever have trouble with dragons here?" asked Kate.

"Sure, we still have a few, and every once in a while a new one will hatch," admitted JoAnn. "Dragons are tough and some of them nearly immortal. But as our people and our processes keep getting better and better, our dragons keep getting smaller and smaller. They have less and less to feed on, as we keep improving."

JoAnn pointed out to Kate that she should not get the idea that the transformation of Normal Medical Center was finished or ever would be. Zapp! was not fixed or absolute, she explained, but a driving force for a journey toward continuous quality improvement and cost containment. Sometimes the road was rough, and sometimes they even slid backwards. But by working together—Zapping together—they were making real progress in three important areas: improving patient care, increasing employees' job satisfaction, and lowering health care costs.

Off to the sides, many parts of the old field were still under construction. In one area, some employees were climbing into a flightworthy *Zapp-craft*. Even the flying craft undoubtedly would evolve into new forms as time went on.

And down a sleek new road from the castle was the landing base for a whole new 12th Dimension fleet—the Ultranormal Fleet. The base looked entirely different from the Normal base because it had been built around an organization-wide strategic plan developed by senior management with input from all parts of the organization. Processes had been developed to provide the best patient care in the most efficient manner. The base had been designed to be an integrated, smoothly running, launching pad for expanding into new health care horizons.

The Ultranormal Fleet, by the way, was commanded by none other than Biff Buffer, and it was managed and operated by many of those individuals who originally had doubted the value—and the power—of Zapp! Now they were off the ground and Zapped on missions of their own. And Flo was flying with them.

Over the years, the Flo-Vision had become as important to Normal Medical Center as standard hospital equipment. At the request of the C.O.O., Flo was no longer nursing full time. She spent part of each day working with a hospital team designed to keep improving the Flo-Vision. In her new role, Flo had the satisfaction of helping *all* the units in the hospital.

All this had taken a long time, JoAnn explained. It had not been easy, but it certainly had been worth it. Not only did people come to work excited about helping patients, they came to work eager to learn more about Zapp!

As they started back, Kate asked, "Zapp! is something I can use in my own job . . . but what do I do first?"

JoAnn was ready for this question because in the years since she and Flo had first learned about Zapp!, lots of people had asked her how they might generate some human lightning of their own.

"Allow me to recommend my Three-step Action Plan for Zapp! Rookies," said JoAnn. "Let's go back to my office, and I'll get you started."

The first thing JoAnn did when they got back from the 12th Dimension was to give Kate a copy of the JoAnn Mode Notebook so that she could study the basic principles of Zapp!

"Here, read this. Start with Step One. I even reread the notebook myself every so often to refresh my memory," said JoAnn.

"OK, but is reading this going to be enough?" Kate asked.

"Probably not," said JoAnn. "That's why I suggest you try Step Two. Come with me."

She took Kate to meet the hospital's staff development director, Claire Burton.

"Kate, meet Claire Burton," said JoAnn. "She's now the hospital's voice for Zapp!"

"Pleased to meet you, Kate," said Claire. "Are you here to get some Zapp! training?"

"Gee, I don't know. Do I really need training?" asked Kate.

"Well, you could learn the skills to improve Zapp! by trial and error, the way I did," said JoAnn. "But that takes a long time, and you can make a lot of unnecessary mistakes. What I recommend is that you build your basic skills in Claire's training programs so that you're more likely to succeed with Zapp! the first time you try."

Kate considered that idea. "Yes, that does sound more efficient."

"And it'll be easier on the old anxiety level," added JoAnn, smiling.

With that, Kate signed up for Claire's introductory program.

Then as she and JoAnn were leaving, Kate asked, "And what's the third step in your Three-step Action Plan for Zapp! Rookies?"

"Don't stop. Keep learning!" said JoAnn.

"What do you mean by that?"

"I mean, once you're on the right path, keep trying, keep improving, keep growing," said JoAnn. "In short, don't stop. Keep learning."

"Well, OK. I'll give it my best," said Kate.

"Good. And if I can be of any more help to you, let me know," offered JoAnn.

"Thanks!" said Kate as they shook hands.

As Kate walked away, JoAnn could almost see the Zapp! beginning to grow inside a new unit leader. And that made her happy because she knew that once Kate saw the power of Zapp!, she'd share it with her department. And once her staff saw the power of Zapp!, they'd share it with their patients.

JoAnn Mode smiled as she realized that's what Flo had been trying to tell her years ago when she first invented the Flo-Vision. Being a health care professional could be exciting. Zapp! could be exciting!

JoAnn glanced down at her well-worn notebook.

JoAnn Mode's Notebook

Three-step Action Plan for Zapp!
Rookies:

1. Read (and reread) the notebook!
2. Get training in Zapp!
3. Don't stop! Keep learning!

As JoAnn turned to walk back to her office, she saw two recently graduated nursing students waiting to talk with her. Immediately, she recognized Sophie and Ron. Sophie was smiling and Ron was grinning from ear to ear.

"Hi, Mrs. Mode!" they both shouted.

"Well, it's Ron and Sophie, two of my favorite nursing students. Congratulations on your graduation from Normal Nursing College. I'm quite proud of both of you," JoAnn said. "What's the occasion for this visit?"

"Well," said Sophie, "we have something to tell you."

"Yes," said Ron. "We've both been accepted as nurses here at Normal Medical Center."

"In fact," Sophie joined in, "our goal is to become as Zapped as the other nurses here at the hospital. This place isn't normal—it's fantastic!"

JoAnn smiled. She wondered if Flo still remembered that first bolt of lightning in the 12th Dimension. She knew that *she* would never forget it.

ACKNOWLEDGMENTS

Zapp! Empowerment in Health Care was truly a collaborative effort in that all four authors played a significant role. The book was based on the best-selling book *Zapp! The Lightning of Empowerment* by William C. Byham and Jeff Cox. Building on this book, Kathy Shomo researched and wrote a great deal of *Zapp! Empowerment in Health Care.* Sharyn Materna, M.H.A., with broad experience in the health care industry both as a medical technologist and a consultant, provided technical expertise and examples.

The named authors, however, represent only a small part of the team involved in producing this book. Many individuals from DDI also made important contributions by critiquing various drafts, offering ideas, and providing real-life examples from their personal experiences; others worked diligently on the production of the book. Individuals who deserve special recognition include David Biber, Andrea Eger, Jill Faircloth, Shelby Gracey, Ken Jennings, Helene Lautman, Anne Maers, and Carol Schuetz. Other DDI associates who assisted with the book include Adyna Akins, Tammy Bercosky, Susan DeLuca, Nena Frederick, Dick Gage, Mike Mariotti, Sherryl Nufer, Cheryl Soukup, Heather Stewart, Mary Szpak, George Updegrove, and Ellen Wellins. Special thanks to Pamela A. Miller and Stacy Rae Zappi for the book's cover design.

In addition, leading health care professionals throughout the United States offered excellent feedback. These reviewers included:

- Joseph F. Constable, Ph.D., Program Director of Health Services Management, Robert Morris College.

- Ellen Gaucher, Senior Associate Director, University of Michigan Hospitals.

- Mary Ann Gruden, R.N., C.S., M.S.N., C.R.N.P., Family Nurse Practitioner, Sewickley Valley Hospital.

- Carrie Hull, R.N., M.S.N.C., Nurse Manager of Medical Critical Care, Butterworth Hospital.

- David J. Jones, M.D., Editor, *American Journal of Medical Quality*.

- Frank V. Murphy, President and Chief Executive Officer, Morton Plant Health System.

- Gregory Nelson, Vice President, The Alliance for Quality in Healthcare^{SM}

- John Paul, Vice President of the Office of Field Services, American Heart Association.

- Sandra G. Stokes, R.N., Consultant/Trainer, University of North Carolina Hospitals.

- Bonnie Wesorick, R.N., M.S.N., President of CPM Resource Center, Butterworth Hospital.

Now that you have read *Zapp! Empowerment in Health Care,* we encourage you to share your thoughts on the book and its application in your hospital. Write to us at Development Dimensions International, World Headquarters—Pittsburgh, 1225 Washington Pike, Bridgeville, PA 15017-2838.

To remind you of the key principles and to help keep Zapp! alive in your organization, Development Dimensions International offers a mug with the key principles and a Zapp! lightning bolt that lights up when hot liquid is put in the cup. Other reminders of Zapp!, such as sweatshirts, T-shirts, paperweights, and pens, are also available.

DDI offers numerous programs to support Zapp!

The Zapp! key principles, the discussion steps, the Action Cycle, and advice on handling particular interactive situations, such as "Taking the Heat," have proven highly effective in hospital settings. They are all integral parts of training programs produced by DDI, which are used by leading health care organizations throughout the world.

The process improvement methods mentioned in the book are proven intervention techniques used by DDI in helping health care organizations become more effective at providing higher-quality health care at lower costs.

DDI offers health care organizations the following programs that are especially adapted to their needs:

- **Taking Action**—This program raises quality awareness and stresses the need for continuous improvement on the job. It builds the skills needed to use the Action Cycle and encourages high involvement to ensure a smooth implementation.

- **InterAction**—This program helps frontline employees develop the skills to work effectively with peers, supervisors, and physicians. It teaches individuals how to build effective work relationships and gain agreement and commitment. Employees learn skills to train and coach others for success, give and receive feedback, influence people with whom they have no position power, and resolve on-the-job conflict.

- **Team Action**—This program builds the skills that all types of teams—including quality improvement teams, project teams, and process improvement teams—need to succeed. Team members and leaders learn skills such as valuing differences, reaching agreement in teams, and participating in and leading meetings.

- **Service Plus**—This program provides the skills needed by customer (patient) contact employees to plan and take actions for improving service. People who regularly participate in telephone discussions and face-to-face interactions with patients learn skills such as meeting and exceeding expectations, handling difficult situations, and planning service improvement initiatives.

- **Interaction Management**—This program is the world's foremost leadership training system for helping first- and second-level leaders create a high-involvement culture. It provides the skills to encourage initiative, foster involvement and collaboration, and coach for enhanced performance. This system offers more than 25 learning units that introduce or strengthen leadership concepts and develop high-involvement skills.

- **Targeted Management**—This program develops specific leadership and management skills, such as developing organizational talent, leading groups toward high-quality decisions, and influencing personal and organizational success. It is best suited for managers and staff professionals.

- **Targeted Selection**—This program trains leaders and team members how to determine critical job requirements, conduct targeted behavioral interviews that assess the job requirements, use simulations to provide additional information, and combine the information in a way that selects the best candidate for the job.

- **Breakthrough Planning**—This strategy and planning session aims your health care organization in the right direction. Based on assessment information, it helps you design a detailed road map to implement Zapp! and continuous improvement.

For more information about Development Dimensions International's training programs or consulting services, call DDI's Marketing Information Center at 800/933-4463 between 8:00 A.M. and 5:00 P.M. EST.